Redeeming Marketplace Medicine

Redeeming Marketplace Medicine

A Theology of Health Care

Abigail Rian Evans

The Pilgrim Press

Cleveland, Ohio

The Pilgrim Press, Cleveland, Ohio
© 1999 by Abigail Rian Evans

From "Chronic Care in America: A 21st Century Challenge," prepared by the Institute for Health and Aging, University of California, San Francisco, for the Robert Wood Johnson Foundation, Princeton, New Jersey, 1996. Reprinted by permission of the Robert Wood Johnson Foundation. • From interviews with Dr. Eric Cassell, Clinical Professor of Public Health, Cornell University Medical College. Reprinted by permission. • Material from Edmund D. Pellegrino, M.D., reprinted by permission of the author. • From interview with Dr. Malcolm Rigler, Withymoor Village Surgery, West Midlands, England. Reprinted by permission. • From address by Ruth Zerner to nurses graduating from Lehman College Department of Nursing. Reprinted by permission.

Biblical quotations are from the New Revised Standard Version of the Bible, © 1989 by the Division of Christian Education of the National Council of the Churches of Christ in the U.S.A., and are used by permission. Adaptations have been made for inclusivity.

Printed in the United States of America on acid-free paper

04   03   02   01   00   99   5   4   3   2   1

Library of Congress Cataloging-in-Publication Data

Evans, Abigail Rian.
    Redeeming marketplace medicine : a theology of health care /
Abigail Rian Evans.
        p.   cm.
    Includes bibliographical references and index.
    ISBN 0-8298-1310-1 (pbk. : alk. paper)
    1. Medicine—Religious aspects—Christianity.   2. Medical care—Moral and ethical aspects.   I. Title.
    BT732.2.E83   1999
    261.5'61—dc21   98-50597
                                                                  CIP

To my dearest children—

Stephen, Nathanael (Nato), Matthew, and

Thomas, and their sister, Rachel,

whose brief life reminds us all of the need for

God's healing power in a broken world

Children are indeed a heritage from God,

the fruit of the womb a reward.

—Psalm 127:3

Contents

Preface

It was during my years as a missionary in Brazil from 1960 to 1967 that I first asked the question, What can the church do besides pray over the dead? We worked in an area where the life expectancy of most people was less than forty years of age. People died of treatable diseases or insufficient food and clean water. This book (along with a companion volume, *The Healing Church: Practical Programs for Health Ministries,* to follow) is an attempt to answer that question.

In my thirty-plus years as a pastor, I found that a good part of my ministry was with those who were sick, those who were suffering, those who had lost loved ones. People hungered not only for comfort and solace but also for the involvement of the church in concrete ways to address their health-related problems. However, a theological foundation is crucial to ground the church's health and healing ministry so that it can offer a theology of wholistic health sorely missing in our society today. This book reflects my own love of the church and the experience of the grace and healing power of Christ in my life. It offers a theology of health, healing, and healers that, I hope, may provide the motivation for the church's involvement in true health care reform.

No author works alone but thrives on the work and insights of many people. I would like to thank the churches I pastored in these past decades who taught me so much about God's grace and healing power. I owe so much to all my family members—to my parents, for their support and love until their deaths several years ago; to Robert, with whom I worked side by side in Brazil; and to John, whose keen intellect has challenged me to clarify my reflections and writing.

I also would like to thank my former colleagues at Columbia University and Georgetown University who taught me about the physician compleat and the ethical quandaries in health care, especially John Downey and Edmund Pellegrino, and my colleagues at Princeton Theological Seminary whose scholarship challenged me to dig deeply into the Bible and a wide range of texts.

Special thanks go to my friend Jan Jacewitz, whose keen reading of the early version of my book helped me to reorganize and clarify my writing; to Janice Miller, my administrative assistant, whose encouragement and excellent production of this manuscript assured its accuracy. I am especially grateful to my research assistant, Jane Ferguson, whose tireless work in locating salient material and critical review of the early drafts of my book enhanced its quality immeasurably. I would also like to mention St. Deiniol's Residential Library in Wales, where I spent several months of my sabbatical in 1996 combing through their wonderful theological collection with the able assistance of their staff.

"I thank my God every time I remember you, constantly praying with joy in every one of my prayers for all of you, because of your sharing in the gospel from the first day until now" (Phil. 1:3–5).

Introduction:
A New Vision of Health Redeems
Marketplace Medicine

The thesis of this book is that the crisis in health care today results from three principal factors: (1) the predominance of the medical model with its reductionism and depersonalization; (2) the rise of corporate-based managed care health systems, which are driven by economics, not patient care; and (3) the failure of systematic health care reform to provide wholistic health care for all. This crisis is exacerbated by society's unwillingness to sacrifice so that all of its members may have their basic health care needs met. The church has the responsibility and the resources to respond to these problems by providing a reconstructionist view of health, healing, and healers. It can recover its historic healing ministry in new and expanded ways, addressing not only sick persons, but also a sick society where justice demands health care reform.

A large number of medical practitioners—for example, Edmund Pellegrino, Robert Lambourne, and William Foege—have recognized the need to expand the medical model and have used language such as "wholistic"[1] and "spiritual" to address the nature of the expansion. Health care professionals as well as the general public are critical of the strictly medical model of health care. Numerous unsuccessful bills have been offered to reform the U.S. health care system, especially in terms of quality and cost. Most of them have ignored the spiritual side of healing. In the United Kingdom we observe a sharp separation between the charismatic and sacramental healing ministries and the medical delivery system. (Though there are notable exceptions discussed elsewhere.)

This book offers an analysis of the contemporary crisis in health care stemming from the predominance of the medical model and the emergence of corporate health care delivery systems. It is divided into three parts. Part 1, "Marketplace Medical Care," examines the ineffective attempts at reforming health care especially by introducing managed care health systems. The failure of health care reform is due not only to political machinations, special interest group agendas, and the complexity of the issues at hand, but most fundamentally to moral weakness and the absence of a cohesive vision of what constitutes an equitable health care system. This lack of shared values for the common good is especially tragic in light of the forty million uninsured in the United States who have limited or no access to basic health care.[2] As well, the moral vision in the United Kingdom following World War II of universal health care is eroding with the growth of private health care and doctors as fund holders.

Managed care health systems have attempted to reform the health care system by reducing excessive medical costs. In this attempt, they further erode the quality of health care without addressing the principal defects of the medical model. Is the cost of health care excessive? For whose benefit should cost-effectiveness be instituted? If savings were achieved, who should receive the money? If health is considered a primary good, is cost a legitimate concern? Is the conversation about health care reform really another way of excluding certain groups of people from health care in the name of saving money?

After chapter 1 raises issues about the need for health care reform, chapter 2 presents the four relevant features and the positive contributions of the medical model. Chapter 3 offers eight general criticisms of the medical model, showing how medical personnel and resources fall short of delivering total health care. Robert Veatch's definition of the medical model is used: (1) the condition of illness is nonvoluntary; (2) illness is equated with organic disease; (3) the class of relevant, technically competent experts is comprised of physicians; and (4) sickness is defined as what falls below some socially defined minimal standard of acceptability. This chapter also examines the narrow definitions of health, healing, and healers that operate within this model.

The reduction of health care to medical treatment results in expensive and inadequate health services. The elimination of spiritual resources and religious beliefs and practices as contributing factors to health reduces our ability to address lifestyle-related illnesses. Yet the medical model has made some important contributions. Its elimination is not advocated, but its integration as part of a more wholistic understanding of health and health care. Health is more than medicine and money, and broader definitions of health help us to appreciate that fact, as explored in chapter 4.

Part 2, "Redeeming Health and Health Care," discusses the need to reform the understanding of health, healing, and healers in order to respond to the criticisms of the medical model and corporate health care. Chapter 5 in this section argues that the Judeo-Christian tradition and its Scriptures provide resources for such a reformed view of health. They provide a positive and visionary direction for dealing with the more systemic issues in health care. The unique aspects of the biblical definition of health are as follows: (1) it is based on a doctrine of man/woman as a unity—both within themselves and with their environment and community; (2) its definition of health as wholeness includes a spiritual dimension; (3) it orients to health instead of sickness; and (4) its primary goal is others' health, not one's own.

This framework shifts the focus from my health to that of others as the driving force in the pursuit of health. Health is viewed in terms of social justice and service for others. That is, one cannot be in full health without sharing the burden of other people's sickness.

Moving from this wider definition of health, chapter 6 examines the concept of healing that is not simply an individual achievement but a community responsibility—a joint venture. Healing from a Christian perspective also embraces suffering; it desires to overcome suffering, however, not seek it. Christ's healing ministry confronted sickness and suffering and taught us about miraculous healing and about how we can be healing agents in a broken world. Chapter 7 analyzes the problematic relationship between faith and healing that arises from Christ's healing ministry.

Part 3, "Healers as Coadventurers in Health," begins in chapter 8 with a look at the central role of the patient as the integrator of the health care team and also as a healer and a teacher. Chapters 9 and 10 explore the roles and relationships of the pastor, physician, and nurse and new models for their cooperation. The book concludes with a call to all of us to be agents of healing in a broken world.

The central themes of the book are the following:

1. Man/woman is an integrated whole—body, mind, and spirit created to live in community.
2. Health and salvation are twin concepts signifying wholeness.
3. Sickness and sin interrelate as a reflection of brokenness (individual and global) but not always in a causal way.
4. Healing includes a wide variety of resources, activities, and attitudes that move us toward wholeness. It may include suffering and is more than curing. It is communal as well as individual.
5. Christ's healing ministry is a paradigm for healing where all resources, including prayer, faith, and medicine, are vehicles used by God, the source of all healing.
6. "Miraculous" healing is not contrary to nature, but a fuller revelation of God's world.
7. Healers are persons who move one toward wholeness—the patient being the central healer assisted by the primary professionals (pastor, physician, and nurse).
8. The church is a corporate expression of an individual Christian's calling to a healing ministry.

These themes, which are rooted in Christian theology, provide a framework for the examination of marketplace medicine and the basis for redeeming health and health care.

Part 1

MARKETPLACE MEDICAL CARE

1

HEALTH CARE IN CRISIS

The crisis in health care is evidenced by the attempts at reform both in the United States and in the United Kingdom. Health care reform was pushed onto the American national agenda for three principal reasons: cost, access, and quality. When President Clinton formed the Health Care Task Force less than a month after his inauguration in 1993, the expectations and excitement were high. The belief was that a piece of legislation as major as Franklin Delano Roosevelt's New Deal was in the making. Those of us who served on the task force were full of optimism that the long-awaited changes in the health care system were under way. Our political naiveté was soon exposed and hard lessons were learned when the health care reform bill never even reached the floor of Congress.

Hindsight, of course, provides many clues about how things could have been done differently by President Clinton's team: more involvement of doctors in drafting the plan; a piecemeal approach to the changes instead of one sweeping bill; less secrecy and more of an open process. Debates raged about a number of decisions: a single payer system versus third-party insurers; the content of the core benefits package; the way in which research would be funded; coverage for mental illness at the same level as for physical illness; methods to pay for the thirty-eight million uninsured while reducing the overall cost of health care.

The Clinton health care debates did put the need for portable health care in the forefront of demands for change in the United States. This paved the way for the Kennedy-Kassebaum bill, which addressed the issue of portable health care. At the close of 1996 this important piece of health care reform legislation was passed by Congress under the title "Improved Availability and Portability of Health Insurance Coverage" and went into effect in July 1997.[1] In essence this bill assured that employees covered under a group health plan for more than twelve months for a medical condition that was diagnosed or treated during the previous six months could not be denied coverage. No new preexisting condition limit could ever be imposed. This applied even if the person changed jobs or health plans. This bill then ended "job lock" by making health coverage portable. The legislation also guaranteed availability of health coverage for small employers. Furthermore, insurance could no longer be denied based on health status, claims experience, genetic information, or disability. In addition, individuals leaving or losing their jobs were guaranteed the availability of individual health coverage when they had had employment-based health coverage for at least eighteen months.

FAILURE OF SYSTEMATIC HEALTH CARE REFORM

Despite the numerous reasons for the Clinton Health Care Reform Bill's failure and the disaster of managed care, there are systematic reasons why health care reform is floundering in the United States and the United Kingdom. The first reason is *moral weakness.* Fundamentally, one must ask, Is health care reform or societal reform needed? Are there sufficient shared values, inclusive behaviors, and communitarian goals? Or do autonomy and individual rights so rule the day that society is not willing to give up a little so that others will have something? Is there a willingness to share? Is a communitarian or even a utilitarian ethic (the greatest good for the greatest number) a possibility, or is this a manifestation of some Darwinian morality of the survival of the fittest? Are justice, equality, and liberty empty ideals, or do they form the basis of health care reform?

The way chosen to care for poor, elderly, and disabled persons is a measure of our moral fiber. What sacrifices are people willing to make for the welfare of others? Health care strikes at the heart of the moral nature of society, as Peter Draper pointed out was the case in England after the war. British society was committed to providing universal health care for all citizens based on the sacrifices they had made during the war. The country had pulled together, and a moral commitment was made to care for everyone. Will Americans rise to the challenge of health care for all? Perhaps the words of Winston Churchill are apt: "You can always count on the Americans to do the right thing—but only after they have tried everything else first."[2] We are now trying everything else.

The second reason that health care reform is not moving forward is the *lack of a consensus.* Bioethicist Madison Powers asserts that the consensus for health care reform is pervasive but shallow.[3] Perhaps there is a shared dissatisfaction rather than a shared vision. Voters in the late 1990s evidenced some willingness to change but to what was not always clear.[4]

Sixty-six percent of Americans named cost as the main problem facing health care in the United States in the 1990s.[5] Among the five health system reform issues suggested, 82 to 84 percent of Americans said being able to choose their own doctor without paying extra and "having access to the latest technology" were most important. More than three-quarters of those surveyed favored providing health insurance through large groups that could bargain with hospitals and doctors for better rates, limiting the prices that doctors, hospitals, and drug companies could charge, and requiring most businesses to pay for employees' basic health insurance.

There was a strong consensus on the importance of comprehensive coverage of health needs so that not just physical but mental illness would be treated and paid for. More than two-thirds favored using government money to provide mental health care to all who need it. In addition, those Americans polled wanted to require insurance companies to provide coverage for chronically ill people at the same price charged for healthy people. On the other hand, less than one-third favored requiring workers who receive health benefits from their employers to pay income tax on the benefits. And almost half said that their support for health care reform would decrease if it increased their taxes.

The third reason that health care change is difficult is the activity of *so many special interest groups,* including the eleven million people who have jobs in the health care industry. Debates also rage between pro-life and pro-choice groups about whether abortion should be in or out of the core benefits package. The effect of pluralism in today's society is to slow down any drastic changes. The United States appears to be a collection of special interest groups lacking a true sense of being a nation.

The fourth reason health care reform is floundering is the *complexity of the issues*—health care needs are vast in scope and are viewed as a fundamental right. How much is really understood about health care costs, patient-physician relationships, or the best health care plans? How does one address an industry in the United States that represents more than $900 billion in expenditures or a medical delivery system in the United Kingdom that is rooted in a government-instituted system?

The last reason that health care reform is ineffective is its *overreliance on the medical model of health care.* This has caused a neglect of preventive health care and the lack of incorporation of complementary health care practices, including spiritual resources and religious beliefs and practices. Rearranging the delivery system rather than changing what is delivered inhibits real change and reform. This reality is clearly observed in the latest U.S. attempt at health care reform under the banner of managed care. Managed care is not systematic reform but supposedly an attempt to control costs. In its first decade, managed care has not succeeded in this goal. Even when there was some reduction of hospital costs, any savings achieved, rather than providing benefits for those who had no health care, filled the bank accounts of health corporation executives or stockholders.

It may be instructive to discuss managed care in some detail to illustrate the need for a fundamental reenvisioning of the health care system. Our assumptions about health, healing, and healers need to be radically changed.

The Rise of Managed Care

Examined in the best light, managed care has operated from three basic ethical principles: beneficence (improve quality); nonmaleficence (reduce harmful care); and justice (decrease the cost of care). Managed health care emerged in the 1990s as an attempt to answer the problem of excessive costs in the U.S. health care system. The hope was that by treating the caring profession as a business rather than a service, bottom-line discipline would bring runaway costs under control. The first question is whether or not commercial principles can be applied to the provision of medical care. The changes in health care delivery are exemplified by the health insurance industry, which created a new method of delivering health care. A wide range of groups emerged to "manage" care, that is, managed care organizations (MCOs), health maintenance organizations (HMOs), preferred provider organizations (PPOs), point of service groups (POSs), independent practice associations (IPAs), insurance reviewers, hospital administrators, institutional managers, and the purchasers of groups needing care who run the health care corporations.[6]

The difference between HMOs and PSOs (provider-sponsored organizations) is ownership. HMOs are usually owned by insurance companies, while PSOs are owned directly by doctors and hospitals. At the end of the 1990s about 14 percent of the nation's more than six hundred licensed HMOs were actually PSOs, according to the Blue Cross/Blue Shield Association. Naturally, the insurance industry tried to keep physicians and hospitals from the lucrative health care market.

HMOs and PSOs both provide medical care to their members for a flat fee regardless of how much care a member uses. To make a profit, they bet that high costs incurred by one member will be offset by the low costs of other members. They risk losing money if their costs exceed their income, so the goal is to exclude persons who are too sick.[7]

Whatever the type, managed health care functions as individual, profit-driven corporations whose product is medical care. The vocabulary used by these organizations reflects their corporate image: the "consumer" (formerly the patient), the "provider" (the physician and other health care professionals), the "insurer" (the reimburser for any care), the "buyer" of health services (most often the large employer organization). A certain dollar amount is negotiated for health care for a certain number of patients whether the care is given or not; the provider shares with the insurer any financial risk for the actual costs of care.[8] And despite the observation by some health industry analysts that managed care heralded an alternative to the medical model, it fits squarely within that model. The managed care system does not attempt to redefine health and sickness but accepts the existing definitions. Exclusion of coverage is based not on new definitions but on cost savings. Managed care differs from the medical model only because it has weakened the authority of physicians by the primacy of the dollar.

To understand the history of managed health care, one must grasp the context in which it first emerged in the early 1930s when physicians controlled the economic power of medicine. In the mid-twentieth century, wealth, power, and trust were given to the doctors. Each year brought better coverage and more treatments. Beginning in the 1970s, there was a breakdown of the payer-provider contract. A resistance to runaway costs developed that gave rise to managed care; in many ways economics changed health care. Patients were billed directly by their doctors an amount that rested largely on the conscience of the physician. If the patient was poor or otherwise burdened, the doctor might waive the bill and increase the amount charged for richer clients. That was called fee-for-service. In most instances, the more medical care delivered, the higher the physician's income; thus, the incentive was for maximum procedures and tests. In its best manifestation, however, the patient's good was primary.

Against this backdrop the first third-party payment system began at Baylor University for public school teachers, a well-organized, identifiable group who could not depend on the charitability of physicians to meet medical costs on modest salaries. Insurance companies began paying teachers' bills, but the amount was still determined by the doctors. As the third-party payment system spread to other sectors of the population, insurance companies gradually dictated to doctors what would be paid for their services. Blue Shield started by covering the costs of surgeons and other hospital-based specialists until it had enrolled fifteen million members in 1950; by 1962 with fifty-six million members, it became Blue Cross/Blue Shield.[9]

Despite this growth, insurance coverage was still spotty and uneven in the early sixties. Twenty-six percent of the population had no health insurance; and only 27 percent of the money that Americans spent on health care was paid for by insurance companies.[10] The average private health care expense of aged persons was 80 percent more than that of the population as a whole, and insurance paid only one-sixth of it.[11]

It is not surprising that insurance coverage was less than satisfactory, given its lackluster record of government support. In the 1940s, Roosevelt deleted the section on health care coverage for the aged from the Social Security Act because of the fear that the Social Security Act itself might fail. National health insurance was uniformly rejected. President Truman advocated health insurance for the aged under the umbrella of Social Security in 1951, which also failed. It was not until 1965, under the Johnson administration, that Medicare for the aged and a Medicaid program for the poor were passed. These initiatives, however, had start-up problems with uneven and incomplete coverage.

In this climate, Henry Kaiser launched what is now the most common type of managed health care system, known as the health maintenance organization, in 1942. HMOs took health insurance a step further by blending insurance and provision of treatment itself. The original prepaid group plans were nonprofit and covered all health needs for a flat monthly fee; money saved from unnecessary procedures was recycled to better preventive care.[12]

However, the growth of managed health care as an industry was practically nonexistent as long as physicians had the economic role and the clout to dominate medicine on the basis of fee-for-service. As insurance companies began wresting economic control away from physicians, they were simultaneously confronted by the alarmingly high increases in the cost of health care exemplified by the medical model.

THE GROWTH OF MANAGED HEALTH CARE

The tremendous growth of managed care in a very short time demonstrates just how profitable the promise of cutting medical costs can be. During the Nixon administration, prepaid group models were transformed into health maintenance organizations. At that point the federal government began helping new HMOs. By the 1980s, many HMOs were profit-making companies.[13] The percentage of the population covered by managed care grew from about 15 percent in 1985 to almost 50 percent in 1995.[14] More than 13 percent of the 38 million Medicare beneficiaries were in HMOs. Congress and the administration wanted to increase Medicare participation in managed care and to offer a broader choice of systems. By 1998, 85 percent of working Americans were covered by managed care[15] and the total number of persons enrolled in HMOs was 70 million.[16] (Note: HMOs are a subset under managed care.) In the 1970s only 6 million people considered managed care an option, prompting one social pundit to note, "This may be the only U.S. industry to go from being considered a communist plot to a capitalist conspiracy in a little over a decade."[17]

Of the 1,500 managed care plans in place in the late 1990s, up to 30 percent of the profits went into the pockets of investors. The total compensation package of a typical managed health care corporate CEO was more than $1 million. Annual salaries built into the packages were also impressive and on the rise. One example was the $3.6 million in salary and bonus paid to Malik Hasan, an entrepreneurial doctor, in 1994. His $5 million or so in stock options was compensation over and above his salary.[18] So attractive was the margin of success that an entire new group of research organizations sprang up around the managed health care field just to monitor it for newcomers or improve the competitive edge for participants. Minnesota-based InterStudy, for example, "maps" the managed care marketplace with research reports that pinpoint HMO enrollment by "product type, penetration, financial measures, premiums and reimbursement methods" in more than three hundred metropolitan statistical areas. The reports sell from a few hundred to thousands of dollars.[19] One cannot help comparing the current entrepreneurial zeal of the managed care field to the market research firms that proliferated in the wake of the technology boom during the go-go years of the seventies.

ASSESSMENT OF MANAGED HEALTH CARE

After an impressive decade of explosive growth that has succeeded in curbing a steep rise in medical costs, managed health care organizations are now on the receiving end of a frontal attack from critics who charge HMOs with nothing less than raping U.S. health care for their own profit. The financial risks for health care costs have been shifted from the insurance company to the physician with incentives to restrain costs. In the last six years the number of doctors has increased by 20 percent, while the number of health care managers has increased by 683 percent in the last fourteen years.[20] The quickest way to make money is to avoid treating sick people.[21] Physicians such as Ronald Glasser, who wrote a scathing critique of managed care, believe that the wellness craze is obscuring the real threat of illness.[22] Balance sheets seem to be the top priority. The applause for the progress of managed care firms may still be ringing on Wall Street, but the needs of the forty million uninsured Americans who cannot afford any form of health care remain unaddressed. Anecdotes abound among HMO enrollees about denial of treatment, limits on hospitalization and choice of physicians, greedy health care plan executives, and a system cutting corners for profit.

Where previously doctors believed it was unethical to advertise, HMOs in the late 1990s competed aggressively for the $80-billion-a-year market, with advertising slogans such as, "You'll feel better with us," and "Be Happy, Be Healthy." Managed care organizations claimed to be primarily interested in patients' welfare, but doctors and patients alike attested otherwise. Most opinion polls in 1996–97 reflected high dissatisfaction by participants in managed care plans. Eighteen percent of *Consumer Reports* readers polled went outside their HMO plan to obtain the care they needed, paying the costs out of pocket.[23] Still, ambiguity predominates when assessing the managed care field in light of the overall state of the nation's health care system. Studies by E. Harris Associates and the Robert Wood Johnson Foundation show that while 53 percent of respondents felt the health care system was getting worse, managed care as a corrective measure got favorable marks from 59 percent of the respondents.[24] However, the poll does not explain what is meant by "good" in the assessment of HMOs. In a September 1998 poll, two-thirds of Americans surveyed said they had some problem with their health care system.[25] However, some flagship health care systems, such as Advocate Health Care, which represents a merger of the United Church of Christ and Lutheran Health Care Systems, are first-rate in their vision for health care and for a more inclusive delivery system. As an integrated delivery system, it can respond more wholistically to people's health needs.

CHANGES IN THE PHYSICIAN–PATIENT RELATIONSHIP

The crucial question that must be asked is whether a health care policy should be cost-driven or care-driven. Who is protecting the traditional ethics of the primacy of patient care? HMOs now talk of lowering the percentage of income that goes for patient care, which is going against everything we believe about health care.[26] Doctors can no longer prescribe what is best for the patient, but only what is covered. Drive-through deliveries, which limited postdelivery hospital stays to twenty-four hours, and the gag rule, which prohibited doctors from mentioning treatment options that were not covered under the patient's HMO, were just the more sensational fallout of the managed care system. An interesting footnote must be added to this practice: Congress passed legislation in 1996 requiring health plans to give new mothers at least two days in the hospital.[27] Some have even quipped that the doctor's office is now known as the insurance company's waiting room.[28]

HMOs pressured doctors to reduce the time allotted to each patient from fifteen to ten minutes. They reward them for "cost-effective medicine"[29] for good reason: one of the problems with the new system is that physicians accustomed to fee-for-service do not know how to do cost-effective patient management. The managed care physician is open to malpractice suits since the system is set up to reward doctors for delay in treatment. In addition, while patients value care by a known physician with whom trust can be developed, patients are forced to relate to a group of doctors. Moreover, doctors can no longer simply refer their patients to the best specialists but must comb through authorized lists to see who is on the list, which may already be outdated.[30] Many doctors spend their time quieting patients' anger at the policies of HMOs. Outside their office door in the hallways, hospital personnel are consumed with conversations about mergers and acquisitions. Patient care seems to be the last item on the agenda.

The patient-physician relationship, the quality of care versus cost containment, patient choice versus organized health care groups—all constitute key ethical conflicts in managed care today. One of the fundamental issues raised by managed care is whether a patient's interests can trump all other needs or whether they should be weighed against competing claims of other patients, payers, society, or even the doctor. The patient does have a fundamental right to participate in sharing the goals and methods of care. The marketplace is not the appropriate arena for patients weakened by illness who cannot defend their rights or negotiate their needs. In fact, now at the end of the twentieth century, a new patient bill of rights and radical reform of managed care are already in process, with more than fifty bills presented.[31]

Older physicians who have practiced under a patient-centered model are especially concerned about the divided loyalties that managed care plans generate, even though these may arise in any contract or covenant relationship. Yet self-interest appears to be rewarded in a way not hitherto seen in the patient-physician relationship. The very structure of managed health care encourages a built-in conflict with the doctor's first obligation to the patient; the good of all the other patients served by the plan and the good of the organization may trump the individual patient's needs. Using corporate terms such as "fund holder" to refer to doctors in the United Kingdom, for example, will begin to shape the reality of who doctors are. When there is a conflict between various obligations, the doctor's first covenant should be with the individual patient who trusts that the doctor will do what is best for his or her health.

It is true, of course, that a physician who accepts employment in a managed care plan incurs an obligation to serve the goals of that organization. In 1998, only 19.9 percent of doctors practiced outside HMOs.[32] However, they are ultimately placed in an ethically untenable position if they cannot meet their primary obligation to the patient. The requirements of the plan could render the doctor powerless to intercede on behalf of the individual patient. Even worse, from the perspective of Edmund Pellegrino, a renowned physician-educator, are incentives and disincentives based on the belief that if all persons serve their own self-interests, the good of the whole will be met. In medicine, the doctor's self-interests, however legitimate, should never be met to the detriment of the patient.[33]

Many observers fear that the role of the physician to protect the good of the patient will be lost in all the debates. As an initial response, forty state legislatures have introduced more than 350 bills to regulate managed care programs; thirty-four of these bills have passed.[34] This points the nation to the red flags that need to be raised about managed health care concerning the quality of care, the speed of care, the qualifications of the doctors, the availability of care, and the cost. The effects of the legislative action will be far-reaching. As a *Time* magazine article pointed out, "managed health care [is] not just cutting costs but changing in a fundamental way how doctors view patients, and perhaps how patients should view their doctors."[35] Doctors become "gatekeepers," determining what specialist services and procedures a patient may receive. Patients become "covered lives" whose health needs are measured by what is reimbursable. Corporate managers decide who gets treated and who does not, based on costs.

Managed care challenges the basic tenets of U.S. medicine—the freedom to choose one's own doctor and the autonomy of physicians to order care as they see fit. Many prominent physicians are afraid that doctors will be reduced to "case managers," "fund holders," or "clinical economists."[36] Primary care physicians become the principal targets for manipulation by managed care because their role is to contain costs. The burden rests with the generalists who as the "ethical gatekeepers" must resist the pressure to become marginal specialists as managed care generally rewards fewer referrals to specialists.

It seems that a doctor can serve the patient's interest only until it conflicts with the managed care plan's guidelines. If the patient's interest holds sway, what happens to cost containment? Reasonable salaries for service rendered should be the practice of physicians; yet their salaries represent more than 18 percent of health care costs in the United States today. As a citizen, the physician is bound to use society's resources wisely and well. Ordering unnecessary tests simply to avoid malpractice suits is not good stewardship. However, requiring advance directives to avoid "unnecessary and futile treatments" because they are not reimbursed was not the intent of living wills. It is true that patients may no longer be pressured by doctors to undergo prolonged testing against their will, but commitment to patient education and choice should not be driven by market concerns.

Another pressing concern is the quality of doctors in HMOs. Are they the best trained, experienced, knowledgeable, and patient-centered doctors available? There is no reason to believe they are better or worse than other certified and licensed physicians since belonging to a managed care plan is more and more the only option for a doctor. Some industry observers have even gone as far to say that credentialing is totally useless. Only 1 percent of the doctors are not recredentialed when evaluations for their continuance with the health care company are done. In fact, the major reason for dropping doctors seems to be their ordering too many procedures or medications for their patients, hence pushing up the cost. This "deselection" process, as it euphemistically is labeled, has become such a threat that new laws providing doctors with hearings in such cases are being considered.[37]

Cost Containment Is a Myth

In assessing the various pros and cons of a managed health care system, one comes to the core question that underlies the raison d'être of HMOs: Do they, in fact, save money? The government reported in 1996 that the rise in health care costs measured in double digits through the early 1990s had shrunk to a 6.4 percent increase. During 1994 there was the slowest growth rate in three years, and costs were expected to grow no more than that in 1995.[38] However, 1998 projections were that health care costs will reach $2.1 trillion—i.e., they will double—by 2007.[39]

Furthermore, 1996 figures indicated that doctors' earnings rose nationally by 6.7 percent, and projections for 1997 and 1998 were that medical care supplies, equipment, and services would increase at 5 to 7 percent annually compared with 2 to 4 percent a year in 1995 and 1996. Health insurance was also projected to increase; however, it is important to note that while HMOs will increase on the average 4 to 10 percent, traditional indemnity insurance will rise by 7 to 15 percent.[40] Yet the savings by HMOs are not being passed on to the patients, who are spending more for out-of-pocket expenses. In 1996 the average person spent $3,759 out of pocket; in 2007 this same person will spend $7,100.[41] Some believe that any savings generated by managed care will go to pay shareholders dividends and not to expand services to the uninsured. (See further discussion on reasons for rising costs at the end of chapter 2.)

The effects of managed care must be watched for possible neglect of persons who already do not have access to health care and for diminished employment opportunities for all health professionals. Adverse selection, risk adjustment, and outcomes measurement as the guiding methods in managed care will result in neglect of persons with chronic illness.[42] There is little doubt that health care companies will continue to increase their profits on an unprecedented basis. Wall Street is bullish on the prospects of health care companies, now that national health reform poses no threat to corporate profits. In 1995, for-profit chain mergers included almost $50 billion in transactions, and three of the largest deals involved Columbia/HCA, which was under investigation during 1997–98 for its questionable practices.[43]

These huge profits might be acceptable if personal health care costs were less. To determine cost-effectiveness of managed care, one must understand how the system works. Doctors are paid in various ways: as employees, as groups of doctors, or through multiplan contracts with multispecialty groups. In one type of plan, physicians receive a salary, but an important part of their income comes from bonuses or other monetary incentives that depend on how well the group does financially. This kind of capitation schema gives doctors incentives to order fewer tests and to defer patient visits; it is the opposite of fee-for-service medicine. With managed care, doctors are paid more for doing less. The system offers perks to physicians for cutting costs, which results in robust profits for the plan and slim treatment for the patients. Corporate cost control means minimizing benefits delivered to members unless they are willing to pay a premium.

Indeed, so "multitiered" is the system that much time is lost on the job for U.S. citizens as they try to navigate the health care system and get reimbursed for benefits given. Causing downtime on the job because of the complexity of the system is only one troubling side effect that makes it difficult to assess the overall cost-effectiveness of managed care. Nurses and other health care professionals may receive pay reductions or even lose their jobs to provide the profit margin for the large corporations. When Marin County General Hospitals in California converted to private hospitals, 540 registered nurses lost their jobs while the hospital reported a profit of $5.6 million.[44] Nurses' and nursing assistants' percentage of annual pay for total hospital costs continued to drop—hovering around $38,000 average annual salary for registered nurses[45]—while hospital CEOs averaged $235,000.[46] One big concern about the impact of managed care is that hospitals will be squeezed so badly they will no longer be able to support research, education, community programs, or free care for the uninsured.[47]

Especially disturbing is the method HMOs use when they do not want to pay for a service. This method is called "rationing by inconvenience"; appeals and grievances go unanswered.[48] This jams the nation's legal dockets, wastes the time of judges, and makes lawyers richer. Based on past experience with HMOs, some believe that managed care does not save money because of the additional costs for multilevel bureaucracy, marketing and advertising costs, and so forth.

Gatekeepers May Not Save Money

Critics of HMOs claim that the gatekeeper general practitioners are costing the health care system millions of dollars because of ineffective office visits and physical therapy. To date there are no clear studies proving that HMOs are more expensive. However, a CAPP Care study shows that gatekeepers increase other primary care and specialist utilization; hence, using gatekeepers may actually be more expensive.[49]

As gatekeepers refer patients to other health care specialists, economics drive some managed care decisions and reward doctors for limiting utilization of specialists. One study by the U.S. General Accounting Office found that little empirical evidence exists on the cost savings of managed care.[50] Premiums for both types of health care plans have been rising at the same rate. Furthermore, some patients' care is better managed by a specialist; for example, advanced rheumatoid arthritis could be more economically managed by a rheumatologist. Some people believe that technology drives costs high. However, for example, if all transplants in the United States were halted, there would be a savings of only $300 million a year, a few hundredths of 1 percent of the total annual health expenditure.[51]

In a 1990 survey of Washington State specialists, 93 percent believed that gatekeeper-based plans would lead to patient dissatisfaction about lack of direct access to specialists; 81 percent predicted that necessary tests would not be performed; and only 7 percent believed that quality of care of the specialists would improve.

"Gatekeeper" may be too adversarial a term because in many cases a general practitioner can manage a problem just fine. The patient does not realize this and thinks he or she needs a specialist. A coordinator can play an important role by overseeing a patient's care. One solution to the financing problems is to also capitate specialists. Thus, the rationing is not simply in the hands of the general practitioners. There certainly seems to be a trend toward reduced hospital days, which is in most instances a cost savings. For example, in California five physician groups alone had reduced the number of hospital days by an average of almost 30 percent from 1990 to 1994.[52]

Another cost-containment measure concerns medications. Drugs are now more often prescribed based solely on whether there is a generic drug or whether a discount is offered by a patient's HMO. Of course, a reduction in drug prescriptions could be good since there is growing literature about fatal drug interactions and addiction to prescription drugs. Nevertheless, drug prescriptions should be based on the patient's good, not on cost.

Mental health benefits have long been curtailed in most health care plans. Of the insured population, including Medicare, 48.7 percent are enrolled in managed behavioral health programs, which is the designation for mental health care.[53] A review of articles about mental health care under the new managed care plans shows that most mental health practitioners say there is poorer care for chronically, seriously mentally ill persons and no care at all for "worried well" persons. For the latter group, the care could prevent them from becoming chronically ill in the first place. Initially, the inclusion of mental health benefits in the Clinton plan core benefits package was assured only when the vice president's wife, Tipper Gore, became an aggressive spokesperson for their importance. In HMOs one sees the use of effective medications, the substitution of day hospitals for residential hospitals, and shorter courses of therapy. The effectiveness of these approaches to mental health care is too soon to call.

Preventive Care Is Offered but Limited

HMOs are supposed to invest in preventive care. Immunization rates at HMOs are high, ranging from 60 to 85 percent of patients needing them. However, HMO businesspersons find that broad preventive care does not pay off in their quarterly and annual bottom-line calculations. Of course, in the long haul preventive care can reduce health care costs.

When routine assessments are made and patients are enrolled in wellness programs, Americans may see managed care at its best. If Blue Cross/Blue Shield Associations added routine, periodic screening for diseases to their coverage, premiums would increase by $7.50 monthly for families. The screening package in many HMOs includes tests for breast, colon, cervical, and lung cancer; heart disease; hypertension; diabetes; thyroid disease; and osteoporosis. Nationally, routine preventive services would add about $3 billion to the nation's health care bill. Under Medicaid all states cover preventive services for children. Nineteen states cover preventive services for adults.[54]

The most important question is this: Is cost containment a moral goal in and of itself if needed health care is expensive? Physicians such as Pellegrino believe their goals are mutually exclusive. Economic constraint is not in and of itself morally justified. Philosophers such as Daniel Callahan would take issue with this analysis. Callahan suggests in *Hard Choices* that allocation of scarce health care resources is a moral act.

In summary, it is not clear that the principal goal of managed care to contain costs has been realized. Stringent cost savings measures have been enacted that may reduce our health care expenditures. However, even a dramatic reduction in costs does not answer the other problems with the medical model, and it does not represent true health care reform.

In the next two chapters, the features and problems of overreliance on allopathic medicine and the need for a radical shift in health care will become apparent.

2

THE FOCUS ON MEDICAL CARE

One of the principal reasons for the contemporary health care crisis is the dominance of the medical model, which conflates health care with medical care. However, that does not mean that the medical model is without its positive aspects. Defining the medical model and analyzing its significant features are important before criticizing it. Both its strengths and its weaknesses should be examined.

FEATURES OF THE MEDICAL MODEL

Medical books and literature do not contain definitions of the medical model per se. Some scholars suggest that the best way to understand it may be to see it in action in a hospital setting.[1] The features of the medical model described here are based on my adaptations of the perspectives of Robert Veatch, Mariam Siegler and Humphry Osmond, and George Engel. Veatch as a religious bioethicist has been writing for decades on the need for medicine to become more patient centered and ethically based. Siegler and Osmond as psychiatrists provide a perspective from inside medicine, and Engel as a medical sociologist provides a more objective perspective. Models are only relatively helpful in explaining operative definitions but at least provide a way of organizing the features of certain phenomena and a means of clustering information for application to a problem or situation. Engel suggests, "A model is nothing more than a belief system utilized to explain natural phenomena, to make sense out of what is puzzling or disturbing."[2] Despite competing models to interpret medical phenomena, the medical model remains the preferred one to describe the reductionistic approach to health care.[3]

Stephen Pattison, a British pastoral theologian and National Health Service consultant, agrees that the medical model dominates the concepts of illness and treatment in today's society. His description of the model is quite similar to Veatch's. He believes that this model concentrates on the body as a machine and on pathology in terms of biology, chemistry, and physics. Illness is any deviation from biological norms, and diseases are believed to be caused by independent entities. Treatment then consists of intervening in the individual's physiology. Scientific research, it is believed, will eventually discover all cures.[4]

Veatch defines the medical model by indicating the relevant characteristics for classifying a negative deviancy within it. In medical terminology, the model serves as a "nosological" device for addressing the concerns of health, healing, and healers. Veatch spells out the characteristics of the model, explains their ambiguities, and suggests that the term be reserved for conditions that most nearly meet the following features: (1) the condition of illness is nonvoluntary; (2) illness is equated with organic disease; (3) physicians are the class of relevant, technically competent experts; and (4) sickness is defined as what falls below some socially defined minimal standard of acceptability.[5]

Illness Is Nonvoluntary and Morally Blameless

The medical model claims that the patient, unlike the sinner or criminal, is not morally responsible or culpable for the condition because illness is nonvoluntary. No longer are all people ostracized automatically as sinners or criminals if they have certain illnesses, as was true as late as the nineteenth century. Although Veatch insists on a distinction between nonvoluntary and nonculpable, these terms may merge as he observes, "It seems clear that one of the primary functions of the medical model is to remove culpability."[6] He then questions whether it is possible to remove responsibility since many illnesses hitherto considered nonculpable have their culpable dimension. For example, cancer has its seven danger signals that a person can detect; failure to do so, for some, indicates culpability. Veatch may incorrectly interpret the medical model as linking the nonvoluntary nature of illness with moral blamelessness and freedom from responsibility for sickness. It is important to distinguish between being responsible and morally culpable; a patient may be responsible for causing her own sickness but still be morally blameless.

It is possible to classify a negative deviance within the medical model as a nonvoluntary illness, without moral blame, while establishing patient responsibility. To illustrate this point, two persons may lead the same dissolute lifestyle—one suffering a heart attack at fifty, the other living illness free until eighty. The heart attack victim did not voluntarily decide to be ill, but his condition might have resulted from earlier lifestyle choices for which he was responsible. However, the fact that he suffered a heart attack, and the other did not, does not make him morally inferior to the other person who outlived him; morally speaking, they receive the same judgment.

The medical model may admit that an illness is caused by a person's lifestyle without relinquishing the description of illness as nonvoluntary. The crucial point is that a patient, unlike a criminal, does not decide to perform an act to bring about a desired state, in this case, illness. For example, a patient may not exercise at all, resulting in the unsought condition of poor circulation and varicose veins. On the other hand, a criminal may buy a gun, go to his would-be-victim's house, and shoot him—all acts that contribute to his original intent, murder.

So a person can perform a voluntary act that results in a nonvoluntary illness, for which that person is responsible. A thirsty person may drink contaminated water, for example, and contract hepatitis. He would be responsible for getting hepatitis if he knew that hepatitis was common in the area, that it was often transmitted in the water, yet he drank the water without first boiling it. He voluntarily set out to drink water, not to get hepatitis. However, he is responsible in part for having contracted the disease because he did not take the necessary precautions to prevent it. Yet this act is not grounds for moral blame.

The recent successful suits against tobacco companies introduce another feature of connecting blame with illness. The absence of warnings about smoking supposedly frees the smoker from blame for her lung cancer. Currently, warning labels on medications may attempt to shift the blame from the manufacturer to the doctor to the patient who uses a drug despite the warnings.

The important point is that in the past some illnesses, such as venereal diseases or alcoholism, carried a moral judgment that the medical model has now removed by labeling them illnesses.[7] However, some patient responsibility is always assumed, even if it is only in the Parsonian sense of an obligation to seek help and to cooperate with the treatment (see later discussion of Talcott Parsons). Furthermore, the legitimacy of exemption from moral and social obligations is relative to a given society. The Victorian woman with the "vapors" was not expected to enter treatment.

The distinction between nonvoluntary and responsible notwithstanding, the perception of illness as nonvoluntary discourages the development of preventive medicine and rehabilitative self-care. If disease attacks an individual outside his or her control, then theoretically, an individual is unable to prevent it by diet, exercise, lifestyle, or spiritual inner peace. Mark Siegler is troubled also that the view of illness as nonvoluntary does not respond to the patient's private concerns about why he or she is ill. This view treats all diseases as if they had natural causes and fails to explain why a particular disease manifests itself in a particular patient. Furthermore, it encourages the denial of symptoms on the part of patients who do not want to acknowledge their illness and are considered removed from its onset.

In summary, the medical model defines illness as nonvoluntary and morally blameless but allows for some degree of patient responsibility for his or her condition as evidenced by the election to seek treatment. However, the focus is shifted from the out-of-control patient to the in-control professional, hence short shrifting preventive medicine.

Illness Is Equated with Organic Disease

Is sickness an objective reality, a subjective state, or a societal construct that exists in the minds of the beholders? In the medical model illness is reduced to organic disease—an entity that invades the body. Disease is defined as a "thing out there" that is now "in here"; health consists of removing that "thing." The assumption is that with enough research, time, money, and information, eventually all disease will be eliminated. Veatch points out the ambiguity of this feature by proposing four stages of subsystem analysis of disease: the deviant behavior itself; the response; the proximal cause; and the ultimate cause. A disease must be clearly organic at all four stages to be classified squarely within the medical model. Often it is difficult to determine the organicity in each stage. Narcotic addiction is organic in some stages and not others, for example, while cystic fibrosis is clearly organic in all four stages.

Veatch concedes, however, that labeling a disease as organic does not preclude its social dimension. Biological aberration is not sufficient for the medical model to classify a person as ill; there is always a socially bestowed negative evaluation of a deviancy to classify it as an illness. Social judgment is a necessary part in labeling the sick. The medical model includes the "sick role" that society assigns to reflect the social aspect of disease. For example, having freckles is a deviancy but not an illness in U.S. culture; possessing them does not qualify for assuming the sick role.[8] The fact that a deviancy is organic is not enough to treat it within the medical model, but its organicity is a minimum requirement. Veatch does not go far enough in his description of this feature, so his description is expanded here to include the medical model's reduction of illness to disease.

Interpreting health and disease primarily in organic terms results in an emphasis on the physical body rather than the whole person—body, mind, and spirit. The patient is viewed as a collection of organs, not an integrated whole. This may leave no room for the social, cultural, spiritual, psychological, and behavioral dimensions of illness.

Engel argues that medicine faces a crisis because it adheres to a concept of disease inadequate to the scientific tasks and social responsibilities of medicine and psychiatry. The medical model is both reductionistic and dualistic in its treatment of illness. Disease is treated as an entity independent of social behavior; all behavioral aberrations are explained solely on the basis of disordered somatic processes.[9] There is no attempt to include other types of symptom clusters. The physician's role as educator and psychotherapist is shortchanged.[10] This is evidenced when physicians may be aware of the sociobiological influences on health and disease, but treat them solely within a narrow medical model;[11] their interest is in the organic manifestations of the disease that qualify a person as sick.

It is important to distinguish between the medical model's labeling of all disease as organic and the false conclusion that hence it is interested only in a person's body. The model's emphasis is on the manifestation of the disease within the body, not claiming that the effects of disease are confined to the body. Side effects of a disease on the whole person may be recognized but relegated to the care of other professionals. For example, a patient's terminal cancer may cause job loss, family breakdown, and severe depression; the physician may recognize these problems as either causing or resulting from the organic condition of cancer, but relegate their treatment to other experts. The crucial point, from the perspective of the medical model, is that the health professional is responsible only for the organic disease, not all of its sociological and psychological side effects.

The Relevant Experts Are Physicians

The medical model insists on a dominant role for the medical profession, especially the physician, to the virtual exclusion of other professionals for the treatment of sickness. Veatch perceives this domination as correct as long as physicians do not attempt to draw all deviancies into their sphere for treatment. Advocates of the medical model, such as Mark Siegler, see its strengths precisely at this point of its physician-centered approach and the resulting patient-physician relationship.

For Siegler and Osmond, the Asclepian authority of the physician underlies the medical model. Once specific individuals are designated as doctors, they are baptized with Asclepian authority.[12] They use this authority to persuade certain people that they are sick and must submit to treatment. This authority, in turn, enables society, vis-à-vis the physician, to suspend societal moral judgments of blame. In the Asclepian paradigm, the sapiential, moral, and charismatic aspects of authority are all interwoven. The sapiential aspect asserts the right to be heard by reason of knowledge or expertness; the moral aspect claims the right to control and direct by reason of the rightness and goodness of the enterprise; the charismatic aspect exercises the right to control and direct by reason (some would say by a God-given grace) especially in response to the shadow of death that hovers over the encounter.

By far the most important feature of this Asclepian authority is the conferral of the sick role.[13] In the absence of this authority, the patient may put the sick role on himself or herself, but without the presence of a physician, self-blame may result. A physician must disentangle the social, cultural, educational, economic, and political factors that brought the patient to the doctor in the first place and determine if any of them are medical ones.[14] This is accomplished through the patient's general case history that fewer physicians may have access to. Since this complaint model of medicine carries the danger of making physicians responsible for responding to all of a patient's complaints, isolating the medical problems and dealing only with them are crucial. At this point assigning the sick role becomes a part of the doctor's authority.

Siegler and Osmond borrow Parsons's definition of the sick role in which persons (1) are exempted from normal social responsibilities by the physician; (2) cannot become ill or get well by an act of will; (3) want to get well as soon as possible; and (4) seek help and cooperate in getting well.[15] In sum, the sick role consists of two interrelated sets of exemptions and obligations: (1) exoneration from certain kinds of responsibility due to illness; and (2) an obligation to seek professional assistance and to get well. The sick role is bestowed as a necessary part of entering what is often a very painful treatment. People may slip in and out of the sick role as their health improves and then fails again.[16] However, in some cases, a patient does not want to leave the sick role, and the doctor must pronounce her or him cured.

The doctor's assignment of the sick role signals to the patient and the world that the illness is an acceptable deviance from normal health. The patient is passive while the physician acts with special authority and power; this asymmetry, far from being negative, enables the best health care to take place. Siegler and Osmond describe the patient-physician relationship in the following way: first, a person voluntarily comes to a hospital or physician; he agrees to be called a "patient" and is referred to as a "case"; he allows a physician to treat him. He is examined in order to discover what he has and not who he is or what he does. The physician prescribes a treatment on the basis of the diagnosis, offering a prognosis. All of this transaction occurs within the context of possible death.[17] Although the physician may assign the sick role, society's definition of health also affects what the physician classifies as sickness within the medical model.

Sickness Is Being Below a Minimal Standard of Acceptability

The medical model, by concentrating on disease, has a limited view of what constitutes sickness; it is any state that falls below an acceptable minimum societal standard of health. Further, it is concerned with a measurable, objective standard rather than a view of sickness as the manifestation of a disease in a particular person. Veatch points out two ways of viewing health: first, as an absolute norm or ideal, and second, as a relative state of healthiness determined by a particular society. According to Veatch, the medical model often settles for a "baseline" definition of health—healthiness rather than health per se. Health is an organic condition of the body that is judged by the social system to be good;[18] it is descriptive rather than normative.

Broad definitions of health, such as that of the World Health Organization, which includes social and cultural conditions, would not be included within the medical model. Health is reduced to the absence of disease or, even more narrowly, the absence of organic disease. Total well-being, whole-person medicine, and spiritual, physical, and emotional health would not be the concerns of the medical model.

In summary, the medical model defines the three major concepts of health, healing, and healers as follows: health is the absence of organic disease signifying wellness; healing is the removal of disease, defect, or malfunction by curing; healers are limited to medically trained professionals.

POSITIVE ASPECTS OF THE MEDICAL MODEL

The medical model provides a useful method for classifying illness and organizing a sickness treatment system as well as creating a way of managing health care. As Veatch states, "A pervasive and complex instrument for interpreting a wide range of behavior, the medical model has served well as a means of organizing our attitudes and actions toward a variety of human abnormalities."[19] He objects not to the medical model per se, but to the ambiguities in its distinctions between voluntary/nonvoluntary and organic/inorganic and to the dangers inherent in its expansionist tendencies. He does not define and describe the medical model with a view to eliminating it. He opposes, rather, its expansion to encompass a widening circle of human variant behavior.[20]

The medical model has its positive aspects as well as its shortcomings. First, it systematically organizes knowledge about health and disease. "The medical model provides a way of organizing and conserving knowledge about disease and its treatment and so enables us to save human lives."[21] With the rapid proliferation of technical information about disease and health prevention techniques it offers necessary rubrics under which professionals can organize as well as interpret and dispense information. The model's systematic approach to disease has enabled tremendous strides in both diagnosis and treatment by harnessing technology and science in the service of medicine.

Second, it provides a system for containing expectations about available health care by limiting treatment to bodily illnesses. Undoubtedly, the World Health Organization's broad definition of health has created unmanageable expectations for health care delivery. By limiting the definition of health, the medical model enables the medical profession to provide specific health care services without being responsible for all of them. There is no doubt that there is an increased number of "worried well," who may need therapeutic services but technically are not ill.[22] Using the medical model as a criterion for treating only certain types of illness means that people can be referred elsewhere.

Some people claim that the medical model has been used in an opposite fashion to classify all aberrant or deviant states, including sin and crime, as forms of illness. Peter Sedgwick calls this inclusiveness "the progressive annexation of not-illness into illness."[23] Many would agree with Sedgwick that the medical model tends to medicalize everything. In the hands of some practitioners it may be used to explain every emotional, mental, and sometimes criminal behavior as having an organic origin. However, if it cannot convert the deviation into bodily terms, it does not attempt to treat it. For example, criminals are sent to prisons, not hospitals, though a merger of this may occur with the "criminally insane," who are treated according to the medical model in psychiatric prison wards. A more interesting case may be the interface with the clergy. Are the demon-possessed thought to have a physical illness, which is mental in origin, or a spiritual illness, which may have physical manifestations? The answer raises the question about who should treat them. (This question will be examined in chapter 5, which discusses the biblical reconstruction of the definitions of illness.) However, this leads to the next positive feature of the medical model.

Third, it has removed the label "sinner" from the sick person; for example, persons who are mentally ill are treated with equal care and concern. Its quest for knowledge of the workings of the human body has provided modern society with the undreamed feats of transplanted body parts, gene therapy, reproductive technologies, and lifesaving treatments that in another age would surely have been called miracles.

Fourth, the medical model operates with an integrated interpretation of health, healing, and healers. It begins by defining health as the absence of organic disease, which forms the basis for viewing healing as the restoration of a disease-free state, and logically results in defining healers as medically trained professionals who eradicate organic disease. The responsibility of these healers is limited to treatment until the disease is manageable. This is a coherent model that has successfully delivered medical care for several decades.

Fifth, through research, experimentation, and scientific treatments, the uniformly fatal diseases of earlier centuries, such as tuberculosis and pneumonia, and childhood diseases, such as scarlet fever, polio, and measles, virtually have been eliminated. One needs only look at the dramatic change of life expectancy in the United States and the United Kingdom to affirm its effectiveness. At the turn of the century a man could expect to live to age thirty-two, a woman to age thirty-five.[24] Today, a man will live to seventy-five, a woman to nearly eighty in the United States,[25] and seventy-four and eighty, respectively, in the United Kingdom.[26]

As the features and strengths of the medical model have been examined, its important contributions are evident. As we move in the next chapter to examine its weaknesses, the goal is not to eliminate the medical model but to develop a collaborative style of health care. This should be built on the significant progress that allopathic medicine has achieved while broadening our understanding of health and health care.

3

PROBLEMS IN THE MEDICAL MODEL

Now that we have acknowledged the importance and contribution of the medical model, we will discuss its shortcomings. The revisionists and critics of this medical model attempt to redefine the three concepts—health, healing, and healers—rather than challenge the coherence of the model. Once the first premise of the medical model is accepted—that health is synonymous with the absence of disease—its definitions of healing and healers naturally follow. Critics note a fraying of the medical model's hard-line definitions by observing that the same treatment can cure some and kill others; that so-called terminally ill patients live for years; that patient self-care may heal where medical treatment fails; that abused bodies resist illness and pampered ones fall sick. They conclude that the neat answers no longer suffice and the very concepts of the medical model must be replaced. Moving from the medical model's strengths to its shortcomings, however, we do well to note that the revisionists and critics fail to provide the kind of integration for their redefined categories of health, healing, and healers that the medical model has achieved.

Criticisms of the medical model cluster around the following themes: (1) the narrow definitions of health and disease limit the scope of healing; (2) the model's expectations of physicians simultaneously expand their authority while restricting their function and excluding other healers; (3) the dominance of physicians and the definition of illness as involuntary render the patient helpless; (4) the reduction of health care to medical treatment results in inadequate health services; (5) the expansionist claims of the model imply a medicalization of most deviancies as well as of society itself; (6) the explosion of available medical technology creates unrealistic expectations; (7) the model produces a kind of medical education in which the technical and scientific override the humanistic and moral; and (8) the type of medical care provided generates exorbitant health care costs. In an analysis of these eight general criticisms of the medical model, the eighth one, exorbitant costs, opened the way to managed health care, as previously analyzed. In subsequent chapters, there will be responses to some of the criticisms of the medical model and managed health care from a Judeo-Christian reconstructionist position.

Healing Is Limited by a Narrow Vision of Health

Some critics believe that by defining health and illness in terms of specific bodily diseases or absence thereof, one creates a dualistic view of human nature and a narrow view of health that limit the scope of healing. Although generally the medical model does not begin with a philosophical definition of health and disease, its operative, underlying premise is that health equals the absence of disease and that illness is any clinically undesirable state. The restoration of health becomes the elimination of disease rather than the treatment of the whole person in her or his setting. Since diseases attack the body, a person's mind and spirit are not of interest. This fragmentation of human nature inhibits complete healing. Furthermore, this disease orientation may narrow treatment only to symptoms rather than to their underlying causes.

Few would argue with the fact that the medical model concentrates on disease rather than health, hence narrowing the vision of health. To a certain degree, it narrowed the definition of health to give physicians something more manageable to achieve. Even Leon Kass, as a physician-philosopher who wishes to broaden the definition of health, admits the need for a clinical focus. Furthermore, if Sedgwick and Pattison argue correctly that disease, health, and treatment are only "social constructs,"[1] then a clinical criterion may be necessary to provide content to the goal of medicine. Pattison broadens tremendously the social dimensions of illness.[2] Sickness is considered a deviant contravention of social norms. What is a disease in one cultural setting can be accepted as normal in another. For example, the Greeks before Hippocrates thought that epilepsy was a sign of divine favor. A South American Indian tribe whose members all have a particular type of skin cancer regarded members who did not have it as deviant. This sociological viewpoint does not provide treatment modalities but is purely descriptive of the definitions of illness. Anthropological definitions of illness also show the hundreds of different ways of viewing illness from one society to the next or even within a society. The cause and effect of illnesses in various societies are understood quite differently. In primitive societies they may be seen as divine intervention or offenses to the "gods."

In addition, there are linguistic descriptions of disease; for example, cancer is seen as all that is evil, and persons with AIDS initially were treated as social outcasts because of society's beliefs about their lifestyle choices, which were viewed as unacceptable by many. However, studies show that people would rather feel guilty about causing their own illnesses than see things as simply arbitrary occurrences.[3]

From this perspective illness and treatment are heavily value laden, and without the medical model to categorize diseases, treatment modalities would be hard to develop. Unfortunately, the medical model's definition becomes either circular, insofar as health and sickness are defined only in relation to each other, or relative to a criterion of wellness in our society. Some critics— for example, Kass—claim that the meaning of health cannot be wholly defined apart from the patient and his or her social role; paraplegia to a physicist may not be as detrimental as an ingrown toenail to a ballerina.

In the medical model's relational view of health, when an individual no longer feels healthy, then one surmises that disease is present. Health and disease are existential concepts. Health is not a part of humankind or a function such as blood circulation, metabolism, hearing, or breathing; it is a by-product of other factors.

Coupled with this relational view of health is the assumption that more medical services ensure a greater measure of health. The National Health Service in Great Britain was founded on this premise, resulting in the classification of problems such as family disorders, attempted suicide, and homosexuality as "diseases," hence medical problems.[4] This perspective produces an engineering approach to health care—the body is a machine to be repaired.

The major impetus to reexamine the reduction of health care to medical care arose from developing countries' substandard health in terms of infant mortality, life expectancy, and prevalence of infectious diseases. Questions emerged whether more medical services would close the gap or whether other nonmedical factors contribute to increased health. A historical review of the facts revealed that the physical and social environment in which people lived and their personal and social lifestyles, such as sanitation, nutrition, housing, education, and communication, were the most important factors that led to a decline in mortality and morbidity in Western countries during the nineteenth and twentieth centuries. Hence, given the scarcity of Western-style medical resources in developing countries, the inevitable question arose whether the distribution of medical services would, in fact, promote the highest level of health.

This view of health as more than the absence of disease led to an acknowledgment of the contribution of numerous disciplines to health[5] and provided the basis for an almost global definition of health. For example, John Snow, M.D., one of the heroes of community medicine, showed that the cholera bacillus was transmitted by polluted water supplies. Hence nontherapeutic and political means were used to address this health problem. The Department of Health and Social Service's report *Inequalities in Health* provides a comprehensive relationship between morbidity and mortality and social and economic structures. The health problem is defined in terms of social equality and justice. The prevention and cure of illness then fit within a much wider political and economic context.[6]

A struggle between the two extremes in defining health—as the absence of disease or the unattainable goal of perfection of body, mind, and spirit—surfaced in the debates over the World Health Organization's formulation. The visionary view as proposed by Brock Chisholm, the then Deputy Minister of National Health in Canada, won the day; it reflected a utopian attitude concerning WHO's mandate. "The world was sick, and the ills from which it was suffering were mainly due to the perversion of man, his inability to live at peace with himself. These psychological evils must be understood in order that a remedy might be prescribed, and the scope of the task before the committee, therefore, knew no bounds."[7] There is nothing wrong with WHO's definition of health as "a state of complete physical, mental, and social well-being and not merely the absence of disease or infirmity"[8] as long as one views it as a goal to be worked on by a variety of professionals and agencies and not as the sole responsibility of the medical profession. A recent illustration of the broadening of the definition of health in the United States is the decision by the Centers for Disease Control to list violence as a health problem.

Daniel Callahan, founder of the Hastings Center for bioethics, argues for replacing the WHO definition because it suggests that medicine can succeed in the goal of achieving complete well-being.[9] Callahan fails to acknowledge, however, that a broad concept of health need not place unreal expectations on the medical professional as long as one does not insist on staying within the medical model for their achievement.

Both the narrow and the broad definitions of health, when applied only to the physician's task, do a disservice to the medical profession. The narrow view reduces the doctor to a body mechanic, and the broad definition places unreal expectations and responsibilities on the physician. One way of reconciling the narrow and broad views of health is to distinguish between the core and the scope of health. The core points largely toward the physiological; the scope broadens out to include social and cultural dimensions. The broader conditions—social, economic, political, moral, and religious—help produce either health or disease.[10]

One solution is to describe health with a qualifying adjective—physical, spiritual, emotional, or mental—and to assign each type of health to a different professional. Alternatively, one could distinguish between cure and care in health care and assign each area to a different discipline. Since technological medicine has become so accomplished at curing infectious diseases and performing surgery, its area would be cure; care would be the responsibility of the pastoral, social service, and counseling professions; and regulation of health care would be handled by legal and political structures. Veatch has proposed

another solution—that the concept of health be relegated to the medical profession and well-being or wholeness be used as the umbrella concept with
health as a subset. Different types of healing and their professionals would
enhance wholeness, but physicians would be responsible for health.
Unfortunately, Veatch's suggestion fails to clarify the link between wholeness
and health and ignores the fact that other resources and professionals, besides
medicine, can promote physical health based on the interaction between
mind, body, and spirit. Furthermore, it does not address the areas of overlap
and how they would be handled (this topic will be explored in chapter 10).

Even if the major role in health care is conceded to physicians, they need
not be judged a failure if they are unable to treat all the sick person's needs.
"The doctor, divinely inspired healer of men, serves also the divine whole by
helping to heal the part."[11] The medical profession's decision to concentrate
on a part of the problem of illness is evidenced by the choice of Asclepius's
logo over that of Hygeia's.[12] Hygeia was the goddess who, around the fifth
century B.C.E., watched over the health of Athens. Her name derives from
the abstract Greek word meaning health (hygiene); her concern was not with
the treatment of the sick but as a guardian of health. Her followers adhered
to the philosophy that living by reason produced health.[13] Progressively, her
cult gave way to that of the healing god, Asclepius. According to Greek leg-
end, he lived in the twelfth century B.C.E., becoming a god in the fifth or
sixth century B.C.E. His powers resided not in living wisely, but in mastering
the use of the knife and knowing the curative virtues of plants.[14] As the god
of medicine, Asclepius overshadowed Hygeia, who was relegated to a sub-
servient role as his daughter (sister or wife) along with Panakeia (all healing),
whose healing powers were employed through the knowledge of drugs.

The myths of Hygeia and Asclepius symbolize a continual oscillation
between two points of view in medicine. On the one hand, health (hygiene)
is viewed as a product of the natural order of things—a positive attribute that
is the result of living wisely; on the other hand, health is understood as the
result of treating disease or correcting imperfections caused by the accidents
of birth or life.[15] Clearly, the medical model emphasizes Asclepius's view of
health. Note, for example, how the school of public health always plays second fiddle to the school of medicine in terms of funding and prestige.

Not only was health narrowly defined, but the rooting of modern science
in the Hippocratic corpus produced a limited definition of disease.
Hippocrates (either mythically or actually) addressed the problems of disease
on the basis of individual clinical observation rather than from any general
theory or speculation. According to the Hippocratic tradition, health and
disease were under the control of natural laws and reflected the influence
exerted by the environment and one's way of life.[16] This contrasted with the
primitive cultures where disease was regarded as the visitation of a hostile

god and with the Hebrew view that illness was the result of sin. The oath's more clinical analysis of disease also provided the basis for a severance between religion and medicine. This view of disease assumed that the body is like a machine attacked by outside forces and its protection depended on intervention by drugs or surgery. This dependency on medical cures produced a heavy reliance on physicians and hospitals, which shaped the whole education of physicians, turning health services into sickness services.

The Hippocratic understanding of disease as an invasive, outside entity led to a dominance of curative rather than rehabilitative and preventive health care. If disease cannot be attacked and eradicated, interest is lost in the patient. "Problems" that cannot be solved—terminally ill and incurable persons—are institutionalized. Death, the worst fate, is to be staved off at all costs. Healing is equated with curing, and caring receives low priority. Some people, neglecting the relative costs of training, interpret the considerably higher salaries of doctors over nurses as a reflection that the cure of disease is more important than the care of patients.[17]

Yet even the critics admit that this disease-attacking treatment model has generated many of modern medicine's successes. Admittedly, bacteria and viruses, gross malfunctions, and accidents are responsible for much of the ill health among populations. However, as we will discuss later, the ten top killers of Americans are heavily affected by lifestyle factors. The fault lies not so much in the relative appropriateness of defining these ills and using medical resources to eliminate them, but in claiming that these ills exhaustively define illness, or that all illness should be treated by medical resources. The corollary to this is that the cure of these invasions takes precedence over other kinds of healing. Health care cannot be conflated with medical care.

Another problem with the medical model's narrow definitions of health and disease is that these definitions are used to classify all nonvoluntary deviancies that are subsequently labeled as purely organic. Is it possible to label any deviancy as purely organic? Veatch suggests that body/soul and somatic/psychological dualism creates difficulty in labeling a deviancy as purely organic. A case in point is narcotic addiction, which is ambiguously organic at all four stages of analysis: behavior, response, proximal, and ultimate cause.[18] Is narcotic addiction, then, a disease or another form of deviancy? Gerald May in *Addiction and Grace* has argued for the systematic definition of addiction that includes physiological, sociological, psychological, and spiritual causes.[19] In fairness, one must concede that not all medical model practitioners convert nonvoluntary deviancies into illness. In fact, some practitioners adhere to a very sharp distinction between illness and other deviancies.

Thomas Szasz supplies a variation on this theme by analyzing the "myth" of mental illness. Nosologies give societies a way of removing deviants from the mainstream; disease becomes a culturally conditioned category claiming to label an isolatable, negative organic phenomenon.[20] In summary, narrowing the definitions of health and sickness reduces healing the whole person—and by extension, society—to curing a disease.

AS PHYSICIAN AUTHORITY EXPANDS, OTHER HEALERS ARE EXCLUDED

From the perspective of the medical model, the physician is the authority and provider of health care. The danger, as Veatch perceives it, is the physicians' extension of their authority from diagnosis to moral judgment to classification, for example, determining if a bump is cancer or a boil, assessing the moral dimension of the cancer, and then deciding whether it fits within the medical model.[21] Instead, Veatch argues that the public at large, or experts in other fields, should decide how to classify a deviancy and who are the relevant experts to treat it; for this reason he asserts that physicians are assessing the moral dimension of disease. This may appear unusual. Once a person visits a physician, the role of a patient is assumed; the physician de facto becomes the appropriate professional. The physician may refer the patient to another professional, but the patient rarely takes the initiative. Furthermore, referrals are almost uniformly to other medical specialists and rarely to another healer such as a pastor. The public needs better education from the medical profession in assessing which problems fall within the medical model and which deviancies are better treated elsewhere.

Of course, there is much conversation of late about changing the physicians' role. One interesting perspective is shared by Dr. Paul Wymer, head of communication and education at the Wellcome Center for Medical Science in England. He describes a new role for the general practitioner as "a local perceiver of social change, an observer of patterns of illness and a teacher and stimulator of imaginative solutions."[22] The physician then would be concerned not only with physical health, but also with cultural vitality, spiritual balance, quality of life, and communal well-being. Oddly enough, as perceptions increase of doctors' ability to control and cure what were a decade or two ago fatal diseases, the public's reaction to them grows more and more adversarial. This attitude is reflected in the increase in malpractice suits. In 1974, 20,000 malpractice claims were brought against doctors each year with an average award of $23,400.[23] A report on medical malpractice litigation by the Rand Corporation's Institute for Civil Justice reveals that malpractice awards have increased from a mean of $1.214 million in 1985–89 to $1.906 million in 1990–95.[24]

Some believe this criticism of physicians, in large part, stems from their own change from servants and caregivers to masters and even demigods. The

fact that they act like God may stem not so much from their supposed control over life-and-death questions as from their belief that they are not
beholden to anyone for their decisions.[25] These criticisms, however, made in
the 1970s and 1980s seem less and less relevant as doctors become employees
of health care conglomerates and may not even be free to prescribe a treatment that they view as medically necessary because it is not covered under the
health plan. In fact, Mark Siegler described the three ages of contemporary
medicine as the "Age of the Doctor" up to 1965; the "Age of the Patient" from
1966 to 1983; and the "Age of the Payer" from 1984 to the present.[26]

Critics might more appropriately question not whether physicians are the
technical experts within the medical model (who else would be?), but whether
only professionals within the medical model can heal or treat patients. Two of
the most important healers may be the pastor and the patient herself. (The
term "pastor" can be replaced in most cases by "priest" or "rabbi" for persons
of other faith traditions.) However, they should work in concert with, not in
isolation from, a physician. One notes in the intensive care unit (ICU) how
the clergy may be sent out of the room while the "real" health care professionals are at work. Furthermore, the medical model often obscures the fact
that politicians, economists, psychologists, educators, social workers, and
family at different times may function as healers. The physician is not the
only health care expert, but is one healer among many.

Even if the concession is made that physicians are the *primary* health care
experts, this fact does not offer blanket approval for everything they do
under the umbrella of medicine. When the physician's function is limited to
technical manipulation and dispensing drugs, the treatment of disease
replaces care of the patient. If no cure is possible, a patient may be abandoned, undercutting the nurturing side of medicine. (Even in nursing, some
believe that the nurturing skills are currently downgraded.)

This contrasts with the turn-of-the-century physician whose only "drug"
was often himself standing by persons with mostly incurable diseases. Lewis
Thomas, renowned physician and author, graphically described his father's
medical practice in this way in the 1920s. When a mother would call at
10:00 P.M. about a sick child with scarlet fever, off Dr. Thomas Sr. would go,
black bag full of placebos in hand, filled with a feeling of helplessness and
discouragement. When, with a sense of failure, he would start to leave after
a two- to three-hour vigil, inevitably the parents would thank him profusely
for all he had done. There was healing—the healing presence of the doctor
himself, based on the family's confidence in him.[27] Although there still exist
these caring doctors who put the patients first, the medical system makes
doing this more and more difficult.

The main criticism of physicians as healers is not *whether* but *how* they
should be the professional healers. The multiplication of specialists hastened

the disappearance of the family doctor (one recognition of this deficit is the creation of the family practice specialty) and an involvement in all aspects of the patient's problems. The specialist concentrates on the disease or malfunction rather than a whole person's interrelated set of needs.

A footnote to this criticism of the physician's expanded authority was discussed under the analysis of managed health care. By making doctors employees, managed health care has curtailed physicians' power as witnessed by the "gag" rule, where HMOs told physicians what treatments they might offer to their patients. (This rule has since been rescinded.) Others within and outside the medical profession claim that the position of the family practitioner as the patient's manager has elevated that specialty; others claim that it reduces it to that of gatekeeper, that is, one who simply approves treatment by the specialists but does not manage the treatment.

PHYSICIAN DOMINANCE RENDERS PATIENTS HELPLESS

The next criticism of the medical model is that the dominance of physicians and the definition of illness as involuntary render the patient helpless. However, before proceeding with this criticism, one word of caution is in order. Although the medical model may exacerbate the helplessness of the patient, illness itself is debilitating; even the "cured" patient is altered by her or his illness. As is true in any field dominated by professionals, the client seeking services is often reduced to a beggar waiting for upturned hands to be filled. The perpetuation of this role by the medical model inhibits and even prevents persons from taking a responsible and active role in their own health care. The impetus to tackle environmental, lifestyle, and work conditions is removed. As people succumb to a medicalization of all their problems, they become more dependent on resources that cannot meet their needs. Patients are viewed not as part of the health team or healers, but as passive recipients of medical treatment. Health is a gift bestowed, not an achievement sought or a responsibility accepted. This is beginning to change with automated patient records so that patients can get second opinions on the Worldwide Web and telemedicine, which puts sophisticated medicine within reach even of persons in the most remote areas.

The medical model perpetuates this passive patient role in two ways. First, the physician dominates in the patient-physician relationship. Since the physician is perceived to be the expert with the necessary information for helping the patient, she takes command of the relationship. Even when the physician attempts to include the patient in the decision-making process, closing the information gap is extremely difficult. The inherent subordination of the patient undermines responsibility and activity. Not only are the patient and physician unequal, but the patient's right to be different or to dissent is restricted in the doctor's office and in the hospital setting.[28]

When people decide to see a doctor or enter the sick role, they often yield their responsibility to help in their own recovery. Generally speaking, individuals weigh information, pass judgments, and struggle with decisions, but in the arena of health care they often throw their minds into neutral or recoil in fear. Accepting the sick role frees patients from certain obligations. The average citizen quarrels more with the president of the United States than with the family doctor. This tendency might appear to contradict the previous point about the current widespread criticism of physicians. Yet a negative appraisal of the profession in general does not extend necessarily to the family doctor. General views about physicians do not preclude adopting a passive role in a relationship with a particular doctor.

However, this passivity within the relationship is now being replaced by leaving the relationship, verified by the increase in malpractice suits. Additionally, patient rights' movements reflect an attempt to "destratify" patients' relationships with doctors and other medical professionals. The Patient Bill of Rights, the Patient Self-Determination Act, and the legalization nationwide of advance directives are evidences of patient empowerment. The change from the term "patient" to "client" or "consumer" further reflects the return of more power to the patient.[29] Despite these changes most critics argue that the patient is still rendered helpless by the dominance of physicians. Even if the physician is not dominant, at minimum he is paternalistic. The problem is not what has happened to the medical profession, but what has happened to us as a result of professional dominance.[30] Changes are needed in the dominance of the physician and the submissiveness of the patient. Ways that this can be achieved will be discussed in chapter 8 in the section on the patient as healer and teacher.

Furthermore, the hospital setting reinforces this professional dominance. It even may foster regression in the patient. The patient is deprived of her clothes, put to bed, forced into a set schedule (including being awakened to take sleeping pills), and judged a good patient if compliant.[31] This isolation, which creates an additional sense of helplessness, is further intensified by removing the person from the community and family milieu. Relatives are too often spectators in the recovery process, and families function as recipients of information rather than partners in the patient's treatment. Even more devastating is the event of death in the hospital. From 1955 to 1967 the number of persons who died in the hospital increased by one-third. The number of patients discharged dead from all U.S. hospitals was 844,000 in 1993, representing 37 percent of all deaths in that year. The entire U.S. population in 1993 was 257,800,000.[32] The patient, rather than being surrounded by family members, is surrounded by machines and strangers. Of course, these statistics may change with reduced hospital stays under managed care, though terminally ill persons still are sent to institutions to die.

An interesting exception to this professional dominance, at least as practiced at Columbia Presbyterian Medical Center, is in the field of rehabilitation medicine. Because a majority of the patients are long-term or even lifetime patients, who alternate between hospital and home, the families are continually involved in treatment and patient care. In fact, patient review committees often make decisions about the next steps of care in light of a family's ability to assist with necessary therapy and care. The rapid increase of chronic illness in the United States and the United Kingdom may make this pattern more widespread.

Coupled with physician dominance, the medical model's emphasis on the nonvoluntary feature of illness further renders the patient helpless. Disease is something whose origin and cure are outside the patient; therefore, the patient is not involved in the process. This passive mode bestowed along with the sick role is one of the medical model's biggest liabilities. Veatch offers several criticisms of defining illness as nonvoluntary: (1) it is reductionistic (since there are other types of nonvoluntary deviancies, there is no need to label them all as illness, for example, stuttering); (2) it fails to account for the discovery of preventable diseases (for example, by genetic counseling, the birth of newborns with congenital disabilities could be reduced; the monitoring of one's diet and lifestyle can reduce the likelihood of a heart attack); and (3) by assigning nonculpability, it removes responsibility, hence challenging patient dignity and autonomy.[33]

The thrust of this criticism may be blunted by maintaining a sharp distinction between nonvoluntary and nonculpable. In other words, just because a disease is nonvoluntary, patient responsibility is not eliminated, as was observed earlier. The principle of double effect applies here: one can choose to work twelve hours a day due to economic necessity, for example, although this act results in unintended illness. The voluntary intention was to work twelve-hour days, but the nonculpable result was to become ill.

HEALTH CARE IS MORE THAN MEDICAL TREATMENT

The reduction of health care to medical treatment may result in inadequate health care services. There are three aspects to this criticism. First, the style or manner of health care delivery is impersonal and dehumanizing. Second, the reliance solely on medical care neglects many vital health needs and resources. Third, elements of modern medical care can in some cases cause illness.

Impersonal Health Care

The operational deficiencies of the medical model produce an insensitivity and depersonalization in health care delivery. Patients shuttled from one specialist to another feel like objects for study, not persons to be healed. There is a lack of primary, preventive, home, and long-term physical and mental health care. Seventy percent of U.S. physicians are specialists compared with 30 to 50 percent in other industrialized countries. The number of general practitioners per 100,000 Americans declined from 83 in 1940 to 32 in 1967. From 1965 to 1970 the percentage of doctors in general practice fell from 22 percent to 15 percent; in recent years only one-fourth of new doctors have gone into primary care. The median income for general practitioners is $93,000 but for a surgeon $200,000.[34]

Too frequently, a given physician may barely know a patient's name, much less anything about his life, dreams, aspirations, or family. On the doctor's grand rounds, a patient's chart receives more attention than the patient herself. Technological medicine, medical-center care, and specialized practitioners are blamed for this dehumanizing style of health care. The emphasis in the last several decades on the need for the study of ethics in medicine is a partial response to this criticism. It questions not the assumption that medical treatment equals health care, but that a more humane type of medical care is needed. This injection of humanism attempts to deal creatively with the tension between efficiency and depersonalization.

Medical Care May Neglect Health Needs

The second aspect of this criticism is more radical, claiming that the reduction of health care to medical care neglects whole areas of a person's health needs. These critics do not suggest that the medical model provides poor health care, is negligent, or is injurious; rather, it is incomplete. In other words, medical care is insufficient in and of itself to realize the maximum possible level of health. The medical model dangerously subsumes all health care under medical care. Poor people in the United States and in the countries of South America highlight that the problem of health transcends the capacities of a medical delivery system. For example, in Brazil in the 1960s, patients with stomachs bloated from malnutrition streamed into the clinics, they coughed from tuberculosis that their systems could not resist, and they were filled with parasites. Although the long-term solutions to these health problems can be viewed as economic and political, not medical, the "health community" needs to address them.

The face of illness has changed dramatically in these past decades. Chronic conditions are the major cause of illness, disability, and death in the United States today.[35] Collectively, chronic conditions account for three out of every four deaths in the United States.[36] For example, an examination of the changing nature of illness and death from 1900 to 1990 revealed a dramatic shift from infectious diseases to heart diseases as the top killers. As medical knowledge has advanced in screening, surgical interventions, and so forth, people with chronic conditions have increased their life expectancy. In addition, the number of elderly persons, that is, those over eighty-five years of age, who are most vulnerable to chronic conditions is significantly increasing; by the year 2000, 13 percent of the population will be sixty-five years or older, and one in eight elderly will be over eighty-four years old.[37]

An important feature of chronic illnesses is that technological medical care cannot meet all the needs of patients with these conditions. Informal caregivers—unpaid family, friends, and community volunteers—provide the vast majority of care and assistance to chronically ill and disabled people.[38] For example, between 1979 and 1990, the number of home health agencies providing Medicare services doubled.[39] Over a similar period (1973 to 1995), the number of nursing home beds per 1,000 persons aged 65 and over dropped from 55.2 to 52.6 and the occupancy of those beds fell from 91.4 percent to 87.4 percent (while the number of nursing homes has decreased by 12.6 percent since 1985).[40]

In addition to the predominance of chronic conditions, according to the Centers for Disease Control, 49 percent of health-contributing factors are lifestyle-related with the other factors being 11 percent medical, human biology 26 percent, and environment 16 percent.[41] People in the United States are no longer dying from infectious diseases in the large numbers that they once did, with the important exceptions of AIDS, tuberculosis, and pneumonia. An analysis of the nature of illness in the United States today is very revealing. The top killers of Americans are heart disease, cancer, cerebrovascular disease (stroke), chronic obstructive pulmonary disease, accidents, pneumonia, diabetes, suicide, cirrhosis, HIV infection, suicide, and homicide.[42] "The six generic risk factors—tobacco, alcohol, injuries, mental health issues, preventive services, and unintended pregnancies—were found to contribute to more than half the deaths and illness in this country. Tobacco was identified as the leading single cause of premature death in the United States."[43] About one thousand premature deaths occur in the United States each day due to tobacco alone. *The Journal of the American Medical Association* reports that the root causes of the top illnesses are tobacco, diet and activity patterns, alcohol, infections, toxic agents, firearms, sexual behavior, motor vehicles, illicit use of drugs, and no access to health care.[44] Teenagers and young adults up to twenty-five years of age die more frequently from existential or spiritual problems than physical disorders. Alcohol-related car accidents, suicide, and homicide are their top killers. As previously cited, violence is now listed as a health problem by the Centers for Disease Control. Teenagers are especially vulnerable to lifestyle-related illness. The 1997 statistics are disturbing:

- Alcohol is the drug most often used by young people, and drinkers are getting younger;
- One in four 10th grade students and one in three 12th grade students report having had five or more drinks on at least one occasion within two weeks of the survey;
- The average age for the first drink is now 15.9 years compared with 17.4 years a decade ago;
- Eight adolescents a day die in alcohol-related car crashes.[45]

In fact, medical care affects only 10 percent of the indices used to measure health status.[46] The microbiologist and experimental pathologist René Dubos, for instance, believed that life expectancy increased more as a result of reduced infant mortality, better nutrition, and sanitary practices than from drugs or medical treatment.[47] Sociologists, such as Rick Carlson, argue that in the future medical care will have even less impact on health: "The end of medicine is not the end of health but the beginning."[48] Since two out of every three deaths in the United States are premature or unnecessary given our technology, lifestyle issues become central. The church has a unique role in addressing lifestyle-related illnesses, which will be discussed in my forthcoming companion volume.

Even persons who accept the centrality of medical treatment in health care are concerned with the technological bent of modern medical treatment. They fear a scienticism, the notion that the scientific point of view holds sway over all other outlooks. Paul Ramsey, one of the leading bioethicists in the 1960s through the 1980s, who died in 1988, described this as the Baconian project that has undermined the contribution of philosophy and religion to the field of medicine.[49] Medicine as an art has disappeared, though this danger has been present for decades. William Osler, the famous physician educator who still impacts the theory of medicine, wrote at the turn of the century, "Medicine is an art, not a trade; a calling not a business; a calling in which the heart will be exercised equally with the head."[50]

An additional concern is that the reduction of health care to medical treatment may eliminate spiritual resources for health and healing. Modern medical technology often relegates religion's contributions to faith healing services. If disease is no longer a result of sin, what does religion have to say about its opposite, health? If a patient has a physician, who needs a pastor? If the hospital is the institution for health care, who needs the church? What can prayer offer that antibiotics do not provide? (It is worth noting, however, that many hospitals have pastoral care departments whose chaplains are viewed as important members of the health care team.) Unfortunately, a dualism results between faith and science, religion and medicine, value and fact, pastor and physician. This neglect of the spiritual resources for health stems not only from the focus on medical care, but also from the narrow definitions of health and disease. (Fortunately, in the late 1990s there has been an emerging interest in the spiritual dimension of health.) If health is defined as achieving freedom from bodily disease, then the spiritual and emotional needs of a person are peripheral.

Another neglected area is health education and promotion. Since doctors must wait for people "to get sick" before they enter the system, opportunities for preventive medicine are rare. Furthermore, health insurance rewards not health education, but disease treatment. The hospital as the primary health institution symbolizes society's emphasis on crisis and reactive medicine rather than wellness and health promotion. HMOs initially attempted to change this by paying for annual physicals, but now doctors and cost-driven treatment plans generally view prevention as a luxury.

Finally, the focus on medical treatment undermines the community as a resource for health care. Generally, we view health as an individual achievement by the physician rather than as a community responsibility. Conversely, illness is viewed as a disease that attacks, not as a result of an unhealthy community. Primitive societies more clearly recognized the interaction between the individual and the community. Although the shaman was designated by the tribe as a healer, his powers always rested with the community, which performed an ongoing role in healing the ill person.[51] They had a period of preparation before the shaman began his work, were present and formed a circle around the ill person, and in some cases were assigned special roles in the healing liturgies. The support of a caring community can facilitate healing in a person's life. This is not to suggest, of course, that the shaman is superior to the modern physician, because the elimination of the superstitions accompanying this style is one of modern medicine's greatest contributions.

Medical Care May Cause Illness

Third, some radical critics charge that medical care not only fails to promote health, but actually causes illness. Medical care is injurious to our health. This criticism relates in part to the side effects of drugs and invasive treatments that ravage the body as well as the psyche. Furthermore, invasive life-extending technologies may prolong the dying rather than enhance the living. Ivan Illich, a Roman Catholic theologian, social scientist, and iconoclast, asserts from a different perspective that the medical model, or more precisely the medical profession, by medicalizing all of society decreases our possibilities for good health.[52] He points to the phenomenon of clinical, social, and cultural iatrogenesis,[53] which results from medicalized health care.[54] In essence, however, Illich's criticism has more to do with the expansionist than with the reductionist tendencies of the medical model.

Dangers of Medicalization Emerge

The expansionist claims of the medical model imply a medicalization of deviancies as well as of society itself. This criticism pertains only if its definition of disease is broadened. In other words, if one of the features of the medical model is that disease is organic, only as that definition of disease is expanded to include nonorganic negative deviancies would medical treatment be used to treat the deviancy. The strict structuralists within the medical model might claim that abandoning the narrow boundaries of the medical model leads to medicalizing everything.

Veatch observes that in a move from a minimal definition of health to an ideal definition, there will be more and more difficulty assimilating this definition, such as the WHO ideal, within the medical model. But if a nonculpable status is assigned to psychological, social, and culturally caused deviancies, one need not classify them as illness or force them into the medical model.[55] In summary, this criticism is applicable only to the medical model if its definition expands to absorb all negative deviancies for medical treatment.

The criticism of the medical model's expansionist claims seems to fly in the face of condemnations of its narrowness. The former critics claim that it makes the narrow represent the broad, in other words, its narrow definitions of health and disease are applied to all deviancies, that is, medicalizing everything. Thus, certain conditions, such as criminal behavior and juvenile delinquency, alcoholism, and heroin addiction, once thought to be examples of personal irresponsibility requiring punishment (including imprisonment), are now thought to be socially induced conditions or organically based illnesses, which can be treated by physicians. All modes of thinking, feeling, and behaving that are considered undesirable, variant, or deviant, as well as general conditions of suffering and disabilities, are to be treated by medicine.[56] This approach does not baptize illness as organic, but subsumes the treatment of all undesirable human conditions under the medical model. As the concept of what qualifies as disease expands, so health becomes a coded way of referring to an individual, social, or cosmic ideal state of affairs. According to James McGilvray, a British writer, this utopian understanding of health as total well-being according to the World Health Organization definition, coupled with equating health care with medical care, has led to the medicalization of society.[57]

Many people question whether prescribing tranquilizers, for example, can qualify as adequate health care for stress-based conditions. Perhaps, instead, this medical approach masks the real causes, inhibiting the identification of the best treatment for these problems. This is well illustrated by a story that Michael Wilson, a British pastoral theologian and physician, tells concerning the appropriate medical response to depression. A group of English physicians in Birmingham, England, were discussing whether tranquilizers should be prescribed for depression following a bereavement. About half the doctors present thought they should be prescribed as a matter of course, and about half disagreed. One psychiatrist offered that if the depression lasted one week, he would prescribe drugs. Another doctor present commented, "I hope you'd let me be depressed for longer than a week if I lost my wife."[58] This story certainly reflects that dispensing tranquilizers might be replaced by referrals to a pastoral counselor or therapist who is better suited to address the heart of the problems facing the man.

The claim that expanded health needs can be met only by doctors is more to blame for the so-called medicalization of society than a crusade by physicians to impose the medical model upon society. Hence, the issue becomes not so much what is classified as illness, but by whom and how it is to be treated. The medicalizing of problems causes our turning to physicians for help in everything from poverty to marriage problems to unanswered prayer rather than doctors volunteering to deal with these problems. When we visit the doctor, she offers what is possible to assuage our suffering, but cannot do everything.

The public's view of physicians is ambivalent. On the one hand, physicians are being criticized for a narrow focus on disease rather than on the whole person; on the other hand, they are accused of too inclusive a view of problems that they perceive should be treated by medical science.

Ivan Illich perhaps best captures society's distrust of the medical model by describing physicians as the new bureaucrats who rule "from womb to tomb."[59] He reflects a basic bias against professionals and Western technology.[60] For Illich, the medicalization of society means that "society has transferred to physicians the exclusive right to determine what constitutes sickness, who is or might become sick, and what shall be done to such people."[61]

To illustrate this, one needs only to think of the medicalization of the birth of a baby.[62] Reproductive technologies have moved birth from a family celebration to a medical event, but that responsibility cannot totally be laid at the feet of the doctors. The mystery of the unborn has also been corrupted into a legal entity. The churches need to face the challenge to clarify the meaning of life as something to be cherished and protected, a meaning that emanates from the Judeo-Christian heritage.

Illich finds the physician-based health care system untenable for three reasons: (1) it produces clinical damage that outweighs its benefits; (2) it obscures political conditions that render society unhealthy; and (3) it detracts from the individual's power for self-healing. Such medical injury does not admit of medical remedies; only a recovery of the will for self-care among the laity and adequate limitations on the monopoly of physicians will reverse the destructive tendencies of the medical model.[63] Medicalized health care becomes an obstacle to the healthy life. For Illich, our basic ability to cope with illness is taken away, our environment is made unhealthy, we are robbed of the meaning of our personal suffering that may accompany illness, and all of these problems are caused by medicine.[64] These factors also lead to the loss of patient initiative in health care.

Illich minces no words. Physicians perpetuate this medicalization as they declare themselves moral arbiters by their designation of the sick role, turning their Asclepian authority into totalitarian power. Even their attempt at preventive medicine by use of the annual physical examination fails because they turn persons into patients before they are sick. Furthermore, exploratory surgery and diagnostic tests hold their own perils.[65] Even worse than their attempts at preventive medicine is physicians' medicalization of terminal care, which places physicians beyond control or criticism. According to Illich, physicians should withdraw when a disease is terminal. Because doctors have usurped all of terminal care, now patients are unwilling to die on their own. All the expectations of very sick patients are focused on science, and patients have become the voyeurs of their own treatment. Even health is no longer ours by native endowment, but an ever-receding goal to which we are entitled by virtue of social justice.

Health ceases to be a natural state as even the normal cycles of a person's life are declared diseases. This is especially true in relation to aging, where little can be done medically, and even pain control is ineffective. Illich will not even credit the medical profession with increasing life expectancy. Instead, he argues, along with others, that this is due to the reduction of infant mortality, which resulted from diet, antiseptics, civil engineering, and the positive value given to children.[66]

Not only health, but the experience of pain, is removed from an individual's control. Increasingly, pain is considered of our making, not a natural or metaphysical evil. Pain is no longer interpreted by the individual but by a third party, most notably the physician who creates a demand from society for painkillers. Pain is something we flee from instead of face, hence its referential aspect is blurred. Questions such as "What is wrong?"; "Why me?"; and "How long?" are never addressed.

Illich laments that society's dependence on the medical profession causes individuals to lose "the healing power in sickness, patience in suffering, and fortitude in the face of death."[67] He calls for a courageous, disciplined, self-critical renunciation of our claim to individual health. We do not have a right to health care that consists of fix-it drugs and high-tech solutions. Illich believes the pursuit of health itself may be futile because humanity will never eliminate pain, will not cure all disorders, and will certainly die. Life cannot be reduced to the survival phase of our immune system.[68]

In summary, Illich carries all the criticisms of the medical model to their extreme; the model, not just its excesses, errs. Illich claims not so much that the medical model is overextending itself, but that it should not exist at all if we want to achieve wholeness as human beings. His analysis parallels the way a Calvinist views sin—the radicalism of human sin is so great that only a complete transformation, a new birth, will restore humanity to what it should be. In the same way, Illich argues, medicine must be thoroughly reborn before health care can achieve its desired state.

Secularists find objectionable Illich's particular Christian perspective, which claims that sickness, suffering, and death have positive aspects; for most people, these are signs of unhealthiness. Illich's presuppositions that healing has a spiritual dimension, that suffering is an occasion for growth, and that death is overcome by eternal life must be accepted before one could agree that these factors are health-giving.

In addition, his dismissal of any benefit from medical treatment overlooks the medical needs of the countries of the Southern Hemisphere. It is ironic that Illich, who trained Latin American radicals at Cuernavaca, should in one sense be so out of touch with one of the greatest needs for revolutionary change—the primitive level of medical care in many areas of the world. Rather than a fear of overmedicalization or the dominance of the medical model, there is in many areas a dearth of all the indicators of minimum medical care: well-trained physicians, knowledge of germ theory, and any facility remotely resembling a modern hospital. More often than not the closest person to a medical professional in remote Latin American interior towns would be the pharmacist.

Parents who have lost two and three children to lack of medical care might long for a little more medicalization. For example, in many parts of Brazil as recently as the 1960s, the lack of nurses necessitated bringing one's own "nurse" in the form of an aunt if one wanted to be admitted to a hospital. Although it is true that the majority of children from developing countries die of malnutrition and parasites rather than operable intestinal obstructions, the absence of sterile hospitals and trained physicians presiding at breech births certainly hinders rather than helps the saving of additional lives.

Illich criticizes medical care in the context of a technological society rather than in the Two-thirds World's crucible of avoidable deaths and unnecessary suffering. His criticisms may be applicable to health care in overmedicalized and professionalized parts of the world, but not in areas that have never seen adequate medical facilities. Of course, Illich would probably respond that the Two-thirds World (or countries of the Southern Hemisphere) is better off without Western medicine, but mortality statistics and the predominance of treatable illnesses would certainly not sustain that conclusion. Such practitioners as psychic surgeons, for example, have killed more people than modern medical practice ever could be accused of harming.[69]

MEDICAL TECHNOLOGY CREATES
UNREALISTIC EXPECTATIONS

Ours is a time of unprecedented medical breakthroughs that create an appetite on the part of the public for every conceivable procedure. So far, the experts and policy makers in Washington have been focusing on the deficiencies and failures of modern medicine: greedy pharmaceutical companies, selfish doctors, government bureaucrats, and ambulance-chasing lawyers. Implicit in their recommendations is the assumption that the elimination of waste will obviate the need for the rationing of health care. It will not.

The greatest part of the increase in health care costs can best be understood as a result not of the failures of medicine but of its successes. Genetic testing to discover cystic fibrosis, cancer, and Alzheimer's disease; gene therapy to treat adenosine deaminase (ADA) deficiency and Lesch-Nyhan (genetic disease where a person self-mutilates); heart and liver transplants; life supports for seventeen-ounce newborns and brain-dead octogenarians—all of these and more are available. Effective medicine does not reduce the percentage of people with illnesses in populations; it increases that percentage. It may seem counterintuitive, but good medicine keeps sick people alive.

People will pay anything to defend against the possibility of death, all the more so when the money involved does not come directly out of their own pockets. The United States is a culture that "wants it all." Medical technology will therefore continue to be expensive simply because it pays for pharmaceutical and other medical supply companies to market a 5 percent improvement of American health even though the refined product might be 100 percent more expensive. This can be seen, for example, in the difference in cost between brand name and generic drugs. One reason for the increase in the overall cost of health care is the oversupply of computerized axial tomography (CAT) and positron emission tomography (PET) scans, as well as cardiac bypass units.

The health care crisis is so severe in the United States because of the preeminent high-technology culture and because of the nature of the American character. Under the medical system in England, health care services are free and widely distributed, but there is a long waiting period for voluntary surgery to correct conditions that are not life-threatening. Americans, on the other hand, would never have the patience to wait for an operation once it was determined to be in their best interest. Consider the struggle in the United States to define such terms as "death with dignity" and "growing old gracefully"; the latter, on closer analysis, means living a long time without aging. Williard Gaylin, a bioethicist who has written about the hard choices that face individuals about health care rationing, believes people in the United States are not willing to give up anything. Dying in one's sleep at age ninety-two after having won three sets of tennis from one's forty-year-old grandson that afternoon and having made love to one's wife twice that same evening—that is about the only scenario Gaylin has found most American men willing to accept as fulfilling their idea of death with dignity. Perhaps standards are out of step with reality. "Instead of debating about regional health alliances and premium caps, one should care about what health services and how many health care dollars should be spent."[70]

MEDICAL EDUCATION NEGLECTS THE HUMANISTIC AND MORAL

The seventh criticism of the medical model is that the model produces a kind of medical education in which the technical and scientific override the humanistic and moral. In the last decade, educators have introduced humanities courses into medical school curricula as a response to the perceived scientism and mechanization of medical education. Prior to 1969, only a handful of medical schools offered courses in ethics and humanities. In 1995 every U.S. medical school taught medical ethics as part of its required curriculum. The traditional model is essentially analytic and emphasizes the process of moral deliberation more than its conclusions. In other words, process takes precedence over content. Alternative models are now developing that emphasize ethical attitudes and moral development, ethical behavior modification, and case study approaches. More courses are including an analysis of everyday ethics, not just sensational cases; teachable moments are also part of the alternative curriculum. Instead of presenting purely hypothetical cases, real patient cases form the basis for discussing the ethical issues.

Major revisions are now being suggested in ethics teaching in medical schools. Students complain that professional socialization undermines their ethical sensitivity and subverts their moral development. The complaint was expressed in the strongest language, as a "process that could dim their idealism, dehumanize them, and lead to 'ethical erosion.'" They desire physician mentors to model ethical decision making and practices in the clinical setting.[71] What is being suggested is incorporating ethics into all four years of medical school. These include virtue-based ethics, narrative ethics, and casuistry along with the principle-based teaching that has dominated since ethics courses began. Interestingly enough, not only moral but spiritual concerns are being introduced into medical school curricula. Since 1994 the National Institute for Healthcare Research, through funding received from the John Templeton Foundation, has supported the development of courses on spirituality at nineteen medical schools.[72]

Whether curricular changes will succeed in humanizing medical education and, ultimately, medicine remains to be seen. The dilemma is that the students' technical expertise may be jeopardized if humanities courses are substituted for some of the science curriculum. If, on the other hand, new courses are simply added, medical education will be unduly lengthened. Moreover, if ethics courses are merely tacked on to already existing curricula, rather than informing the entire educational philosophy, they will effect only minor change.

Courses in whole-person medicine are needed that deal with expanded notions of health, healing, and healers—the cooperation of medicine with other disciplines. Changes in the entire philosophy of medical school education are necessary, emphasizing patient-centered medicine, preventive care, and a wholistic understanding of health. The current pattern of studying cadavers before operating on live patients, and racing through clinical rounds with an eye to exotic diseases rather than everyday suffering persons, must be changed if future physicians are expected to be ethically sensitive and service oriented. Without the proper education it is difficult to move from an objective and detached analysis of disease to a compassionate and caring concern for ill people.

Who gains admission to medical school in the first place is at least as important as what is taught. Since to a large extent a student's value system and worldview form before entry into medical school, who the student is upon entrance will determine to a large degree the future doctor. The ever-expanding expectations of the amount of knowledge that must be mastered by physicians mandate against accepting medical school applicants who rank high on values and service orientation, and low on academic indicators. As well, the majority of applicants and accepted students to medical schools are science majors. Almost 74 percent nationally of the applicants to medical school in 1980 majored in science, and during the decade that followed this number continued to increase.[73] This means little exposure to humanities courses in the undergraduate years. Some attribute the lack of studying humanities to the concern over grade point average (GPA). "Some [premed students] deliberately choose not to take courses in the humanities which otherwise interest them, precisely because they fear not obtaining the obligatory 'A' grade."[74] Arts and humanities are perceived to be unrelated to the practice of medicine.

According to several studies, medical school admissions committees weigh scientific attitudes more than any other factor.[75] This may have its roots in the Flexner Report, which placed a heavy emphasis on the knowledge of science as a prerequisite for admissions. Prior to the Flexner Report in 1910, there were no standards for doctors, and formal scientific education was not required. Abraham Flexner, a U.S. educator and founder of the Institute for Advanced Study in Princeton, New Jersey, revolutionized and narrowed medical education with his report. The medical profession was in disarray, and Flexner's job was to address the problem. Flexner was single-minded in his appeal to the knowledge of chemistry, biology, and physics as the only basis for admission to "a really modern medical school," brushing off the acquisition of any nonscientific preparation to "a varied and enlarging cultural experience."[76] The result was the disappearance of almost all alternative medical systems and practices.

In the past few years, however, some questions have been raised about the validity of this heavy emphasis on the sciences as adequate preparation for medical school. Reports suggest that undergraduate courses in humanities and studies in bioethics, philosophy of health care, and other nonscience courses in medical school may, in fact, produce more humanistically oriented physicians without jeopardizing their scientific expertise. A study at the State University of New York at Buffalo revealed no significant difference between the medical school GPAs of science and nonscience undergraduate majors. The basis of the study was a statistical analysis of grades in the first two years of medical school, clinical performances in the third year, and National Board Medical Examination (NBME) scores.[77]

An additional study, cited by the same authors and performed by Harrison G. Gough, concluded that science students achieved higher GPAs in their first two years of medical school, but by the fourth year of medical school were indistinguishable from their nonscience undergraduate classmates. Others claim that Medical College Admission Tests (MCATs) and GPAs have little relationship to future performance as a physician; hence, even if science majors did better in science subjects, an undue emphasis on a science background would not be justified.[78]

Along these same lines, a study of the class of 1982 at the College of Physicians and Surgeons at Columbia University showed no significant correlation between the number of undergraduate humanities or science courses and MCAT and NBME scores. However, the number of math courses appeared to significantly improve MCAT scores.[79]

These studies illustrate that even by academic measurements undergraduate humanities courses need not be sacrificed for the sake of science. If we continue to admit students to medical schools with purely scientific training, reorienting them with a few ethics courses will be difficult. Of course, data are still unavailable to prove a correlation between the study of humanities and more ethical behavior. One study done at the College of Physicians and Surgeons at Columbia University did, however, show a positive relationship between the study of humanities and involvement in service and religious collegiate activities as well as the possession of certain moral attributes and ethical sensitivity.[80]

Accepting and training students on the basis of the medical model will perpetuate a technical and scientific medical education. Critics of the medical model say the most effective way to change its dominance is at the level of medical education. The face of medicine could be changed if humanities majors with a strong service orientation were admitted to medical school, and the curriculum itself embraced a strong emphasis on values, humanities, and whole-person medicine, with public service an integral part of the student's medical education.[81] Additionally, if theology students were trained in health care, the resources for health care would be dramatically enlarged. Clinical Pastoral Education (CPE) programs in seminaries began in the 1960s as a way to expose theology students to the clinical hospital setting. These programs can exacerbate a continued reliance on the medical model of health care. They place students in a crisis-centered hospital setting where primary health care and preventive medicine are not part of the context of their work. However, it is true that theology students have received a good introduction to death and dying issues. Parish-based CPE is a partial response to that criticism by removing it from a medical crisis setting and putting students in local churches.

There may be some changes in medical education if physicians such as Malcolm Rigler can broaden their influence on the way health care is practiced. His medical practice in Birmingham, England, uses visual images, storytelling, poetry, and even drama to dispel low self-esteem and promote a healthier lifestyle in his patients. Artists, writers, musicians, and actors have all visited his health care clinic over the past few years to perform or to work on projects with local people. Rigler stated,

> The arts have a role to play in at least two ways. The first can be a form of art therapy, where through making things or doing things or creating something, a person can gain a degree of confidence in their own ability to do something positive. Then the arts, through photography and writing and video work and so on, can take pictures, or make pictures with words, and help the community see where people are in different situations, which will eventually affect the medical practice.[82]

Dr. Wymer commented on the effect of this innovation where art teachers and students from a nearby school helped make a CD-ROM to educate patients about asthma. School students described it as a revolutionary approach to health care and the learning of science.[83] However, despite encouraging signs of more wholistically oriented doctors, the typical medical student is more commonly interested in medical technology and the biosciences.

MEDICAL CARE COSTS SKYROCKET

The last criticism of the medical model is that it generates exorbitant health care costs. The accuracy of this criticism is difficult to assess without an in-depth analysis of comparative costs between the medical model and alternate models of health care. Such analysis is outside the purview of this book. Nevertheless, a description of medical model costs is valuable to depict statistically the patterns of spending and the extent of the crisis in U.S. health care in the 1990s.

Health care expenditures in the United States totaled $949.4 billion in 1994 and comprised 13.7 percent of the gross domestic product, a dramatic leap from the $26.9 billion, or 5.1 percent of GDP, the nation spent for health in 1960, according to the U.S. Census.[84] Consumers spent $488.1 billion, or 51 percent of the total. Of that amount, consumers paid $174.8 billion in out-of-pocket expenses for health services and supplies while another $313.3 billion was spent for insurance premiums (this amount covers benefits and amounts retained by insurance companies for expenses, additions to reserves, and profits).

The government accounted for $420.8 billion, or 44 percent of the $949.4 billion sum. Most of the government expenses—fully 72.1 percent—were federal, with Medicare topping the list at $169.2 billion, followed by Workers' Compensation at $18.9 billion, and Defense Department hospital and medical care at $13.1 billion. Other government expenses included maternal and child health care programs, medical vocational rehabilitation, and medical research. The remaining 5 percent of the $949.4 billion total included privately funded construction.

Hospital care claimed the largest personal health care expenditure for both consumers and the government at $338.5 billion, while physician services came in second at $189.4 billion, and drugs the third highest expenditure at $78.6 billion. In descending order of amount the 1994 data show that nursing home care cost $72.3 billion; the net cost of insurance and administration (including expenses of federally financed health programs) was $58.7 billion; a total of $49.6 billion was spent for private nurses, podiatrists, optometrists, physical therapists, clinical psychologists, chiropractors, naturopaths, and Christian Science practitioners; dental services cost $42.2 billion; home health care accounted for $26.2 billion; and "medical durables" such as eyeglasses, hearing aids, wheelchairs, and crutches cost $13.1 billion. It should be noted, however, that these figures have recently changed, as annual expenditures decreased, for example, for the hospital component from 3.0 percent in 1994 to 2.4 percent in 1997 and for the doctor component from 2.5 percent to 2.0 percent in the same period.[85]

Another interesting aspect of health care spending is the number of Americans with chronic conditions and their impact on cost. In 1995 there were 99 million persons with chronic conditions, representing a cost of $470 billion. By the year 2010 that will increase to 120 million persons at a cost of $582 billion.[86]

On a personal level, an American family paid on the average $1,742 for health care in 1980. The cost had climbed to $7,797 in 1993. By the year

2000, it will double to more than $14,000 annually. If health costs had risen with the rate of inflation from 1980 to 1992, each American family would have had $12,000 more in personal savings.[87] Consider that on a national level U.S. automakers now spend more on health care for their employees than they do on steel! Health care added $1,100 to the price of each car made in the United States in 1992, double the amount it added to Japanese imports.[88] Our present health care system is slowly but surely putting our nation out of business on the international market.

The irony is that all of these billions of dollars dedicated to the health care industry have not even delivered heath care to many Americans. Despite sky-rocketing expenditures, there were still 40,582,000 uninsured Americans in 1997 who received little or no health care.[89] Critics of the medical model contend that medical care expenditures correlate poorly with health levels in a community. At base, the medical industry seems to be the only beneficiary of the country's medical care debacle. With the growth of Medicare and Medicaid, hospitals began controlling more and more of health care since doctors could no longer carry their equipment in little black bags. Today, the world's largest for-profit hospitals, based in the United States, have annual revenues exceeding $10 billion. This amount translates to a tidy income for hospital administrators and doctors on the corporate executive staff, insurance companies, prescription drug manufacturers, and medical equipment and supplies vendors, who basically control both profit and nonprofit hospitals. That health care is big business is evidenced by the number of U.S. health care administrators, who are growing at a rate four times as fast as the number of U.S. doctors. One hospital reported having 3,200 different types of accounts receivable.[90]

A legitimate question is, What is the real picture of health care costs? Obviously, large health care costs are not simply the result of the medical model. In 1990 the U.S. government was responsible for 41.6 percent of health care costs, which included medical research, construction of hospitals, Medicare, and Medicaid. During the 1970–1990 period, the increase in health care costs was attributed to inflation, population growth and an aging population, and technological advances.[91] However, determining whether health care costs are increasing in real dollars and as a total percentage of the gross national product is a bit more problematic in today's shifting managed care climate. The runaway costs of 1970–1993, when real per capita health spending growth was just below 5 percent, dropped to 1.5 percent per capita for 1993–96. The projections indicate spending will increase again to 3.4 percent between 1997 and 2007.[92] However, total health spending will increase from 13.6 percent of the GNP in 1996 to 16.6 percent of the GNP in 2007. It is still unclear whether managed care will restrain the costs of use of emerging medical technologies, but it is clear that managed care has reduced hospital costs. (In 1990, average per capita health care expenditures for hospital costs were 9.4 percent and in 1997, 2.4 percent.)[93]

Continuous pressure by the public and the medical community for hospitals and physicians to acquire the *very* latest technology adds to the cost. In a conversation in the early 1980s with Dr. Elizabeth McSherry, Veterans Administration Hospital physician, she cited that the price of one CAT scanner, for example, equals the annual salary of twenty hospital chaplains or a whole department of physical therapists. Furthermore, expensive tests are routinely run by medical professionals as self-protection from malpractice suits. The sad truth is that Americans are not getting the kind of health care they would expect from the amount of money they are spending for it. Especially in light of the fact that the United States ranks twenty-first out of twenty-four in infant mortality worldwide, and ranks sixteenth for women and seventeenth for men in life expectancy, high expenditure does not equal high-quality health care.[94]

Numerous studies emphasize the need for extensive national reform. A 1996 *Consumer Reports* series estimated that a combination of overpriced and unnecessary treatments and a large health care bureaucracy were creating $200 billion a year in excess costs.[95] Health care costs are fast outstripping our ability to pay. Changes are drastically needed in the type and method of future health care. Given our current patterns of health care, both cost containment and "everything for the patient" cannot be achieved. The American way of health care is fast disappearing with unlimited tests, treatments on demand, multiple specialists, high-tech procedures, long hospital stays, and unrestricted choice of doctors. This situation has given rise to managed health care as one approach to reform, as discussed in chapter 1.

This does not mean that health care systems abroad are without their problems. Although the United Kingdom has been a shining example of nationalized medicine in the past, about one in four British citizens now has private health insurance. So inadequate is the system that some predict that the nationalized service is in danger of becoming a social orphan, serving as a last resort for the poor. In 1995–96 the National Health Service (NHS) spent $33,481,000 for health care in England. (The U.K. population is 58.4 million compared to 248,709,873 in the U.S.)[96] Surprising to some, physicians are considered self-employed and are contracted by the state. Very few physicians exclusively practice privately, but BUPA, one of the United Kingdom's private health companies, has established a private primary health care service. In 1998, 5.85 percent of the U.K. gross national product was spent by the NHS and 1.02 percent of the GNP for private health care.[97]

Under the leadership of Margaret Thatcher and Kenneth Clarke, Minister for Health, in the late 1980s, economic competition and the doctor as fund holder were introduced into the NHS by way of the Government White

Paper of 1989 entitled "Working for Patients." The main points of the paper were hospitals' ability to become self-governing, general practitioners controlling the budget for patient services, and providers competing for patients.[98] It is too early to assess if the NHS is moving to an economically driven system, but it is true that there is a two-tier system where patients of fund-holding general practitioners receive treatment sooner than non-fund holders. It now appears with the Labour Party's victory that fund holding may be phased out. However, the impact of the 1997 Government White Paper, "Designed to Care," is not known at this time.

The level of satisfaction with their health care among the British people is hard to assess. By contrast, Canada, which spends about 9 percent of its GNP on health care,[99] boasts a satisfied citizenry, who say they almost never have any difficulty getting treatment for financial reasons; in a recent poll, 7 percent of Americans said they did.[100] Many people look to the Canadian model as one of the best.

This extensive critique of the medical model is not meant to suggest that this model should be eliminated. Instead, medicine should take its place alongside the full health care armamentarium. The miracles of technological medicine are truly amazing, but it should not become a new god. Health and health care are more than medicine and money.

4

Health as More Than Medicine

and Money

The discussion about the medicalization of health care and the failure of systematic health care reform introduces the broader question of what is meant by the term "health." The baseline definition from the medical model's perspective is simply the absence of disease. Clearly, "health" represents more, but how much more? Should it be viewed as a virtue or as a responsibility? Should it be given eschatological significance? Should health be treated in social, geophysical, or even cosmic terms?

The following summarizes some of the more creative (but somewhat esoteric) ways of looking at health. Each has value in that it further expands our concept of health and thus provides a basis for a more productive understanding of healing and healers. This chapter will look at health as a value, a virtue, the primary goal, or one among many goals.

Health as a Value

First, is health seen as a value in every society? It is clear that the answer depends on how it is defined. Physician-scholar Edmund Pellegrino suggests a variety of ways in which health functions as a value: subjectively, as interpreted by society; objectively, in terms of scientific and personal factors; and most important, normatively, as a moral value. For him, it is not an absolute but a conditional value except in the context of medical practice.

As a positive concept, health is close to the Greek ideal of harmony between the varied components of our organism and life situation; health becomes a major means for the improvement of human existence. Or as Galen expressed it, health is that state where we are unimpaired in doing the things we wish to do.[1] Greek medicine and philosophy's definition of health reflects its view of life's goals as well-being and happiness. Democritus, for one, by using the principle of harmony or balance, believed that the maintenance of the calm of the body was equal to health or well-being (*eukrasia*), and the calm of the soul (*sophrosune*) to happiness.[2]

The following questions should be considered in discussing health as a value or a goal: (1) Is it a positive value? (2) Is it the primary goal of human existence? (3) Is it the most important goal for any individual? (4) If health is a value and a goal, does it also signal and entail the presence of virtue, or is health itself a virtue? The way in which these questions are answered, of course, depends on one's definition of health. Those who agree that health is a virtue, a goal to be possessed, and the absolute goal of human existence generally define health as wholeness. On the other hand, those who limit its meaning to physical health accept that it is one of the goals of life, but not the ultimate goal. For the secularist and the Christian, health as a goal means two different things. Health can be a value without being the *summum bonum*.

Part of the debate about health as a value rests on the distinction between the normative and the descriptive positions. Strong normativists believe health judgments are purely valuative, while weak normativists perceive them as descriptive as well as normative.[3] Dubos regards health and happiness not as absolute and permanent values, but as constituting biological and social adaptation: "Health and happiness are the expression of the manner in which the individual responds and adapts to the challenges that he meets in everyday life."[4]

In Greek philosophy, for example, Aristotle taught that health was a subset under happiness—one of its components. Does this mean one cannot be happy without being healthy? Perhaps in the sense of absolute happiness, yes, though *eudaimonia* for Aristotle was contemplation—an intellectual activity, not a bodily one. He defined health as "the excellence of the body; a condition which allows us, while keeping free from disease, to have the use of our bodies."[5]

Wholeness entails not only an internal integration, but also a harmony with our environment. The Russian philosopher Prince V. F. Odoyevski (1803–64) used *tselmost* (wholeness), the whole person in the whole society in the whole reality of his environment.[6] We might even say that "health is the milieu (human and environmental) which enables people individually and socially to grow towards fullness of life."[7] The milieu for creating health begins with the molecule, then the cell, the organ of the body, the whole body, the family, the community, the country, and the cosmos. Health takes on a global or cosmic dimension and means a restoration to wholeness. However, even though health is influenced by the whole of life, one needs to focus on the particular factor at any given time that is needed to promote health.[8]

HEALTH AS A VIRTUE

Ivan Illich, the iconoclast theologian, takes a slightly different tack. He claims that health has been made largely impossible today from a technical point of view.[9] From Illich's perspective, the pursuit of health is a selfish one. In his usual overstatement, he claims that in the last fifteen years, propaganda supporting hypochondria may have reduced smoking and butter consumption among the rich, and increased their jogging, but not changed the technological destruction of U.S. society and the medicalization of health and society.[10]

The concept of individual human life has been replaced by the generic concept of life. A person has now been reduced to an immune system, and health is a measure of the immune system's fitness for living. From the descriptive perspective, disease is malfunctioning. Health is whatever works in a satisfactory method.[11] Disease relates to a whole range of categories of deviant behavior.[12] Health and disease draw their meaning from the culture. The integration of social, cultural, and economic resources is influenced by one's community and country.

If health is a value, is it also a virtue? If there is no responsibility for health, it cannot be a virtue. Although Englehardt, for example, identifies values in both health and disease, health reduces to an aesthetic concept akin to beauty rather than to virtue.[13] Kass questions that equation: "And while poor health may weaken our efforts, good health alone is an insufficient condition or sign of a worthy human life."[14] Kass disagrees that the norms of health and disease correspond to values such as happiness and well-being: "Health is different from pleasure, happiness, civil peace and order, virtue, wisdom, and truth."[15] Happiness (pleasure) is not an appropriate goal of medicine. Other nontherapeutic endeavors, including abortion, cosmetic surgery, social adjustment, obedience, or development of moral virtue, should not be viewed as goals of medicine.[16] (Some people, of course, might disagree that these are nontherapeutic.) This line of argument rests on the limitation of health to a physical state. From this perspective, health generally is one among several goals, but not the primary or sole aim of human existence.

Another aspect of defining health is deciding whether it is an absolute or relative value, or both. The principle "that it is good to be healthy" functions as a moral absolute. Health is selected as a prime value before any particular interpretation of it. However, health is not always the highest value, but simply the highest value within the context of the medical decision; only in that context does it take precedence over other values. (Pellegrino denies the claim that he makes health the primary and absolute value.) It can be either a relative or an absolute value depending on the decision-making context. It is a relative value in relation to other societal values such as jobs, national defense, housing, and so forth. It is an absolute value in relation to programs designed to achieve health.[17] In other words, when someone lacks health and seeks assistance in obtaining it, it becomes an absolute value both for the person who promises to heal and for the one who needs to be healed.

Health then is an absolute value within the medical context; it functions as a normative concept in medicine. In turn, the principle "that it is good to be healthy" functions as a norm in medical decisions.[18] However, other values, such as the rights of the patient, her or his professional and personal autonomy, should also be weighed.[19] Health then is a fundamental value, that is, always taken into consideration, but when necessary can be laid aside for other values. Health is both an ethical and a biological value—an ethical value because it is a good chosen by persons; a biological value because it is desirable for the body.

In summary, health can be conceived as a value in a variety of ways: (1) a social good; (2) an absolute intrinsic need; (3) a state of affairs extrinsically valued; (4) a state of affairs intrinsically valued; (5) a criterion for comparative judgments or statements of fact; (6) a scientific concept; and (7) a combination of all of the preceding modulated by social, cultural, and historical valuations and disvaluations.[20] Despite all these ways of understanding health as a value, the most important is recognizing health as a moral value.

HEALTH AS WELL-WORKING

There are several aspects to the definition of health as well-working and well-being: unity of the person; internal and external integration of a person with his or her world; excellent functioning; wellness; and moral goodness. Well-working is broader than wellness, whose only goal is a sanitized rather than a healthy society. "Wellness" is a clinical word that contrasts with disease. Admittedly, some writers such as Halbert Dunn use the term to refer to an integrated or harmonious interaction of body, mind, and spirit, but that appears to stretch its meaning. Authors such as Parsons apply "well-working" to somatic health and define it as a state of optimum capacity for the effective performance of valued tasks.[21] For others, health signifies more than proper functioning—a general well-being. Health means capability, vigor, and freedom; a strength for life; the integration of the organs for the exercise of psychophysical functions. "Health is the strength to be as man."[22] The Institute of Religion and Health reflects this same view of health: "[Health is] found in a man or woman whose living reflects a sound and liberated mind, body, and spirit, freed in a healing community to have integrity, to love, and to work for good."[23] (In this schema, sickness then is defined as disorganization and crisis.)

Well-working may include the development of the basic unity of a person. That unity does not come automatically. "Health is not the lack of divergent trends in our bodily or mental or spiritual life, but the power to keep them together. Healing is the act of reuniting them after the disruption of their unity. 'Heal the sick' means help them regain their lost unity."[24]

This approach to health considers the individual, her innate genetic limitations, the environment in which she must function, and the final outcome of the interactions of her body, mind, and spirit.[25] Health equals the well-working of the organism as a whole or how the body functions according to its specific excellences.

For a naturalist such as Christopher Boorse, well-working may entail doing what is typical of a species design, that is, conformity to the excellence in a species design.[26] The normal is natural, that is, healthy. "The normal . . . is objectively and properly, to be defined as that which functions in accordance with its design."[27] Health concerns both physiological and functional normality. The latter is an important part of physiological health for two reasons: (1) people want to pursue goals where physiological functions are isolated; and (2) physical health contributes to all kinds of activities.[28] This theoretical analysis of health is value free and relates not to the whole of the person, but to the performance of each part in its natural function.

In this context, well-working means wholeness in action. The well-working body is the one that achieves the norm between excess and deficiency (shades of Aristotle's definition of virtue as the golden mean). For this reason, doctors should attend not only to the cure of disease, but also to health, wholeness, and well-working. Health in this sense is a state of which one is barely conscious. "The healthier we feel, the less we take notice of it and know about it. We do not think of the effortless expenditure of negative impulse, and we use our resources as the need arises in the environment and society in which we are placed."[29]

For others, the concept of well-working is extended to include one's relationship to his or her environment. Optimal health is not a condition of an individual, but a state of interaction between a basically hostile environment and a series of natural and developed defenses. The homeostatic balance of forces is the goal; this balance may be accomplished by decreasing the threat of the environment or by raising the capability of the host to defend herself. This partially reflects what René Dubos means by health as more than a biochemical state, but a social functioning—"the ability to adapt to stress."[30]

Bernard Martin comments, "The healed man, therefore, is a man in whom the obstacles to the development of his true nature have been eliminated."[31] The healthy person possesses a feeling of joy and strength. Without knowing how it all happens, without any sensation of his organs, he lives with a natural urge to develop and express himself.[32] This "medicine of the person" (a term Paul Tournier coined in 1940) is not just medical healing but the restoration of a person to her true destiny. Finally, health as well-working implies patient involvement in the healing process. We are responsible for our own state of health; our way of life becomes very important, a state of affairs that has implications for the role of the patient as healer.[33]

One wonders who has the authority to define illness and health. The medical profession has been allowed to co-opt their definitions, and theology has been largely excluded from this discussion. As Pattison suggests, the church in its healing ministries has an opportunity to engage in these critical discussions but has often failed to do so.

HEALTH AS A THEOLOGICAL CONSTRUCT

From a theological perspective health is not a static concept; it is linked to enabling the full health of others. A "vital criterion" of Christian health care that emerged from the World Council of Churches' Christian Medical Commission in 1982 was concern for "those who are not cared for and to whom no prestige is attached."[34] Health is the outcome of justice in which all people have access to health care. The commission overwhelmingly favored an integrated definition of health care. "At the core of healing is a restoration of unity" in the understanding of health as the integration of body, mind, and spirit. This original biblical understanding of integration may have become compromised by the influence of Greek philosophy with its separation of body and soul.[35] "We still act as though salvation is concerned with the individual's soul and healing with the individual's body," the commission lamented.[36] In its widest sense, the commission agreed, "health is a dynamic state of well-being of the individual and of the society; of physical, mental, spiritual, economic, political and social well-being, in harmony with each other, with the material environment and with God."[37]

Pattison and others within the British perspective criticize this theological translation of health as wholeness as a pie-in-the-sky approach to illness and healing that is unconnected with reality. They want to draw people away from some kind of idealistic harmony and consensus. This seems rather surprising, for without a vision of the future one can hardly hope to bring about transformation. Furthermore, according to David Hilton, former associate director of the Christian Medical Commission of the World Council of Churches, a broad vision of health may move society to change its current nonsystem of health care. Hilton, who worked for years as a medical missionary in Africa and who currently is a consultant to churches on congregational health ministries, notes that since the surgeon general has been reporting for years that more than 80 percent of our sickness is preventable, an approach focusing on helping people stay well might be a more reasonable alternative to a sickness system. A system is needed where health promotion and prevention are at the center of our vision.[38]

Various Christian writers offer different definitions of health. According to Morris Maddocks, the goal of one's health is to be healthy for God, but also to enjoy health for its own sake.[39] For Michael Wilson, as love, beauty, and joy contain a foretaste of the wholeness in God's realm, so does health.[40] For Denis Duncan, health is both a property and a quality of life; it is a means, not an end. Here it becomes an instrumental not a primary value; that is, one may need to sacrifice one's health for someone else's gain. Duncan refers to "holy harmony" as the definition of true health.[41] Health is the functional integration of these constituent elements. A healthy person is one in whom all obstacles to the development of his or her true nature have been eliminated.[42]

The broader definitions of health just reviewed have opened the way for a reconstructionist interpretation of health and sickness. Some of them have been embraced by health care professionals as they struggle to meet the health needs of the whole patient. The groundwork has been established in part 1 of the book as we move toward reframing health and health care.

Part 2

Redeeming Health and Health Care

5

REENVISIONING HEALTH
AND SICKNESS

Part 1 identified some shortcomings and problems in the medical model and managed health care that have produced a crisis in health care. These have led to a reductionistic view of health, which some have attempted to broaden. A radical reconstruction of the understanding of healing and healers is needed, therefore, to respond to the criticisms of the medical model and the shortcomings of managed health care. The Judeo-Christian tradition and its Scriptures provide a positive and visionary direction for dealing with the more systemic problems in health care and can thus serve as a base point for any such reconstruction.

The previous definitions of health as well-working, a value, and a goal foreshadow the biblical understanding of health as wholeness.[1] Is there anything in the biblical definition of health as wholeness that is not included in a discussion of health as well-working and well-being or as a goal and a value? The unique aspects of the biblical definition of health are as follows: (1) it is based on a doctrine of humankind as a unity—both within us and with our environment and community; (2) its definitions of health as wholeness and of sickness as brokenness include a spiritual dimension; (3) it orients to health instead of sickness; (4) its primary goal is others' health, not our own; (5) it broadens healing to include any activity that moves us toward wholeness; and (6) it understands healers as persons who move us toward healing. These aspects provide the foundation for a radically different understanding of health care.

A WHOLISTIC VIEW OF HUMANKIND IS KEY

The human being is a paradox: an angel and an animal; a poet and a tyrant; a saint and a sinner. We are more than the sum of our parts. We are in the process of becoming—both essence and existence. We are normal or abnormal, sane or mad, healthy or sick, successful or unsuccessful.

The biblical definitions of health and sickness derive from the view that the human being is a whole—body, mind, and spirit—made in God's image, created to live in relationship with God and others. "May the God of peace sanctify you entirely; and may your spirit and soul and body be kept sound" (1 Thess. 5:23). In contrast to the medical model and its revisionists, the Judeo-Christian perspective starts with human beings and how their nature determines the meanings of health and sickness.[2] Its view of human nature affects the definitions of health and sickness, and of healing and healers.

There is a reciprocal relationship among the three parts of human nature. Christian theology teaches that the immaterial soul during a person's life unites to the material body in an indissoluble, substantial unity. It has an analogical relation to the union of the human and divine nature in Jesus Christ.[3] The inseparability of that union can be observed in the influence of the parts on one another. One's heredity (germinal plasm) may influence the development of mental life. Physical changes may result from mental processes, for example, blush, pallor, cold sweat, partly through physiological or pathological occurrence. Mental changes may be provoked by physical states of a physiological or pathological nature, for example, menstruation side effects in some women.

It is a grave error to elevate one of the three parts over the others. This tendency is especially prevalent in medicine, but apparently is not just a contemporary problem. Plato believed that the great error of his day in the treatment of the human body was that physicians separated the soul from the body.[4] Healing is based on respecting all aspects of our nature. Modern specialists have succeeded in taking Humpty-Dumpty apart, but the challenge to the contemporary healing professions is putting him back together again.

Instead of splitting human nature into parts, one should view it as a unity of body, mind, and spirit;[5] the connectedness and indivisibility of the whole person.[6] The human being as a psychosomatic unity is an established scientific fact. Health, in one sense, consists in holding these parts together in vital equilibrium. The body identifies us with basic animal impulses, but also serves as the "temple of the Holy Spirit." The mind centers both instinct and impulse and reflective and creative powers. Mental states may predispose persons to illness as well as release vital forces in preventing sickness. The spirit enables us to transcend ourselves and our world. "The human spirit is the place where faith, hope, love, and laughter are born and nurtured."[7]

Despite the importance of acknowledging the unity of a person, it is possible for one "part" of a person to be healthy and another not. At any given time, attention may focus on one aspect or another, responding to the need presented. For example, a person's organs may be functioning well, but emotional and spiritual health are neglected. However, eventually a mental/emotional/spiritual malaise may affect the body; optimum health is achieved only by inner and outer harmony.[8]

A contemporary analysis of human nature eradicates the spiritual aspect or at best relegates it to the theologians. The Hebrew attitude toward human personality was very different from the Greek dualistic understanding. The Hebrew term *nephesh* meant "principle of life." So man/woman is a body animated by this "principle of life." There was no immortality of the soul, or immortality of the *nephesh*. Another word used was *rûach,* a type of divine inbreathing. This spirit means breath, life, wind, vital principle of life, or source. The human spirit pervades every aspect of one's nature unlike the Greek concept of a soul, which is a distinct and discrete part. There is a profound sense of the unity of humankind that comes from the sense of the unity of God. Jesus laid hold of this integrated view of persons in his own healing ministry.

Psychology and psychiatry occasionally show an interest in our spiritual side. For example, Erik Erikson's view of the centrality of the problem of identity[9] and the psychiatrist's critiques of Cartesian dualism move beyond a mere material view of human nature. However, psychology seeks to replace dualism with a psychobiological view rather than reintegrating the spiritual aspect.[10]

How can we understand the spiritual side of our nature and define spiritual well-being? As Craig Ellison points out, behavioral scientists have avoided the study of spiritual health and disease because it seems impossible to develop any objective definitions for the purposes of measurement and analysis.[11] The National Interfaith Coalition on Aging helps in some measure with this definition: "Spiritual well-being is the affirmation of life in a relationship with God, self, community and environment that nurtures and celebrates wholeness."[12] Spiritual well-being is two-faceted—relationship with God and inner unity and satisfaction about one's self-identity and purpose—and both elements are transcendent.

The spiritual nature motivates and enables us to search for meaning and purpose in life and provides an integrative force in relation to the mind and body. The spirit affects, and is affected by, a person's physical state, feelings, thoughts, and relationships. Spiritual courage, for example, may enable people to transcend physical disabilities and suffering and to interpret them within the context of a deeper positive meaning.[13]

Ellison provides a helpful distinction between spiritual well-being and spiritual health and maturity; spiritual well-being is the outward manifestation of an inner state. This distinction frees one from the need to measure the inner contours of one's spirit. Further, it acknowledges that newborn Christians, for example, may not reflect all the "fruits of the Spirit" (Gal. 5), but will begin to realize a certain degree of spiritual well-being. The concept of maturity in Greek (*teleios*) means full development, purpose, aim, or desired state. *Teleios* is related to the idea of wholeness—a goal that one moves toward, rather than a state that one has attained.

Granted that health is wholeness—a goal that one moves toward—then is being healthy equal to being human? Is one more completely human, the healthier one is? The answer depends on the definition of health. If it simply equals physical well-being, the answer is certainly no. However, if health is the integration of all aspects of one's being, then being healthy reflects all each person was meant to be. There is a restlessness about life, a struggle to move toward completion, a yearning for something better. In these terms, total health is never reached and only briefly enjoyed. From a theological perspective, health is an eschatological idea, that is, what God promises and offers in the end. We do not know completely what health is because we have not totally enjoyed it.

With a vision of what we should be, we are confronted with what we are—broken and imperfect. From the Judeo-Christian perspective, although originally whole, now we are broken. Our image is distorted, a reflection in a cracked mirror. In theological language, we label this brokenness. In the Hebrew it is *shabar* (broken, fractured) or *abad* (broken, destroyed), and in the Greek, *hamartia* (to miss the mark). We have a tendency toward evil, but we have the capacity to do what is good. This recognition that we are not all we could be is crucial to our subsequent understanding of health. If one is broken, if all of one's parts do not work in harmony, then perfect health will never be possible because the impediment is within the person. Hence one disease is simply replaced by another.

A distinction, however, must be made between brokenness of form and of action. It is possible to achieve wholeness of action if not form. Here we see another way in which health and salvation relate because sanctification as well is a movement toward wholeness. Jesus Christ's obedient acceptance of death on the cross was perfect action, even though the form, that is, his body, was wounded and bleeding.[14] Similarly, a person may have a poorly functioning body, for example, be unable to walk, but may have an integrated worldview.

Given this perspective, is wholeness of mind and spirit more desirable than wholeness of body? In one sense, it would seem to be more desirable. For the Christian, maturity of spirit enables one to surpass the limitations of body and mind, while maturity of body does not equip one to overcome the brokenness of spirit and mind. Spiritual maturity also may be possessed by a child whose simple faith in God and people enables a clarity of vision that gives strength in the face of physical disease and suffering. (Remember Christ's admonition to become as little children.) The danger in a hierarchy of our three aspects is that, from the perspective of Christian theology, although mind and spirit are perfected and continue into eternity, the body is also transformed and resurrected; all of the parts are valued in God's sight as essential to the continuity of what constitutes an individual.

If one argues that human nature is imperfect, to what extent is it broken? The Reformed tradition, rooted in Augustine, emphasized our total depravity. An alternative tradition, such as Manichaeanism, insisted that the physical laws of nature and sin ruled one's bodily life, while one's mind or soul might rise above nature and relate itself to God. This view created a dichotomy whereby the church cared for the soul and medicine cared for the body. Salvation and health became two separate goals. Still further, the Roman Catholic perspective, rooted in Thomas Aquinas's natural law theory, had a more positive view of human nature as well as of the unity of mind and body.

The theological perspective of human beings as broken should not be confused with a deterministic view of human nature. The theories of behavior that have dominated much of modern psychiatry limit our movement toward health. Szasz in *The Myth of Mental Illness* gives us a clear analysis of the results of applying the principle of physical determinism to human nature.[15] Historical events, that is, genetic-psychological factors, become a determinant of future human actions. This view precludes explanations of valuation, voice, and responsibility in human affairs. From the biblical perspective, we are free and responsible agents in regard to the natural order and other people. Richard M. Hare, a contemporary philosopher, has joined others in teaching that freedom and reason are central to being a moral agent.

Analyzing human beings in relation to their three-part nature is not sufficient for understanding the full Judeo-Christian perspective. We should be viewed in relation to our environment—as social beings. We are defined not only by our internal workings but also by our social relationships. The life situation of each person provides a context for understanding who she is. The community health movement has recognized this social matrix and sought to respect it by organizing interdisciplinary health teams of social workers and social scientists.

John Dolan and William Adams-Smith, writing about the impact of philosophy on medicine, point out the importance of seeing ourselves as part of nature as well as of our culture. They believe that this change in philosophy, carrying with it, as it does, the realization that we are part of nature and change with it rather than being detached observers, is the single most significant factor in contemporary medical history. The obvious effect of this change has been an increasing social awareness of the problems of population control, aging, and the cost of restoration and maintenance of good health.[16] Western society has too long neglected the communal dimension of human nature.

Especially from the Jewish perspective, seeing men and women as part of the community, that is, the nation of Israel, was crucial to understanding who they were. Carried into the Christian tradition, this communal dimension of our nature is reflected in the image of the church as the body of Christ. (See Ephesians 4, Romans 12, and 1 Corinthians 12.)

Psychologically, this understanding of human nature has important implications. People are made to be in relationship, experience acceptance by others, and find a meaning and purpose in life outside themselves. This orientation toward others is a vital part of what it means to be healthy and to actively participate in moving toward health.

HEALTH AS WHOLENESS RELATES TO SALVATION

Defining health as wholeness is not unique to the Judeo-Christian perspective. Etymologically, "whole" is rooted in the Old Slavic word for "complete" and the Old Prussian and Middle High German for "health" (*heil*). The classical Greek word *hygeia* stands for the Indo-European *Sugwiges,* meaning "living well" or "well way of living." According to Kass, the Greek word for health is not related to all the words for healing.[17] However, in the Greek of the Christian Scriptures, to heal and to save are synonymous; since heal means to make whole and wholeness equals salvation, they are interrelated. Kass is referring to the fact that the two branches of medicine in the classical Greek tradition—health and hygiene—were totally separate from each other.

Absence of Disease versus Wholeness

The parable of Jesus' healing of the ten people with leprosy captures the distinction between health as the absence of disease and health as wholeness. All ten were healed of their leprosy. Nine went on their way and missed their chance for psychological and spiritual transformation. One of them took the opportunity to stay behind and accept Jesus' deeper healing. Christ said to him, "Your faith has made you well" (Luke 17:19).

In biblical language, wholeness is *shalom*—not only inner unity but also outer social harmony. Hence the societal, relational, and spiritual dimensions of life all presuppose and relate to one another. "*Shalom* is not something that can be objectified and set apart. It is not something which can be enjoyed in isolation. *Shalom* is a social happening, an event in interpersonal relations. It has to be found and worked out in actual situations."[18] *Shalom* represents bodily health, contentedness, good relations, and so forth, which happen when God's will is done. One must experience peace with God before one can know the peace of God (Rom. 5; Eph. 2).

The Judeo-Christian framework shifts the focus from personal health to that of others as the driving force in the pursuit of health. Health is viewed in terms of social justice and service for others. One only is whole who is joined to the suffering of others. In other words, one cannot be in full health without sharing the burdens of others' sickness. Wholeness is not solely an individual achievement but, in part, a joint adventure.[19]

Other definitions of health tend to be "I" oriented, what is experienced and achievable for the individual. Health in the biblical context is other-directed. For example, Christ's health suffered while he was making others healthier; Dietrich Bonhoeffer described Jesus as "the man for others." The desert fathers risked their physical health, by giving up the necessities of life, to witness to the centrality of Christ in their lives. The journey to wholeness may entail some brokenness. Ironically, as others' health becomes the primary goal, personal health may improve; it becomes a by-product of this other-directed orientation. This is a different communitarian ethic where the individual is not lost but the good of the whole is desired.

A word of caution is in order. This approach is based not on an aesthetic disregard for the body (the body is the temple of the Holy Spirit), but on a higher regard for others. Furthermore, Jesus enjoined us to love our neighbor as ourselves as an important check against self-abasement and hatred.

Another significant contribution of the biblical perspective is its focus on health rather than disease. The creation story in Genesis spells out the original nature and intention of man and woman—to be God's children and to enjoy God, each other, and the world. This story gives us a vision of what we were meant to be. The description of the Fall introduces sickness as a distortion of that wholeness, but contains a promise of how we can move toward the restoration of that wholeness.

How Health and Salvation Relate
The unique dimension of the biblical understanding of health as wholeness can be determined by examining its relationship to the twin concept of salvation. Health and salvation are both parts of God's plan for human wholeness. Physical healing *may* be a sign of God's saving care.[20] Too often we reduce health to bodily well-being and confine salvation to the state of the soul. In the Bible no such dualism exists. The doctrine of God's incarnation in Jesus Christ helps clarify the Christian understanding of the relation between health and salvation. The incarnation requires an expanded notion of humankind and calls for the integration of body and spirit.

Early Christians had to fight the Gnostic influences of their day, which regarded the body as evil and required its denial in an ascetic ethic. Gnostics repudiated the reality of Jesus' incarnation and denigrated the bodily nature. The apostle Paul, who fought the Gnostic point of view, recognized the importance of a person's total being when he referred to the body as the "temple of the Holy Spirit" (1 Cor. 6:19). Paul's doctrine of the resurrection of the body reflected an understanding of salvation that addressed and comprehended the whole person (1 Cor. 15:35–58).

Some argue from the Christian perspective that life and physical health are not the greatest blessings. Although obedience to God may bring happiness, health, and prosperity ("But strive first for the realm of God and God's right-eousness, and all these things will be given to you as well" [Matt. 6:33]), the cross ultimately transcends these lesser goods: "Those who lose their life for my sake will find it" (Matt. 10:39).[21] A person may be a sound specimen in body and quick of mind, but "lost" in the sense of the Christian values of living. "Health and sickness, therefore, are not the conditions of greatest concern to Christians. What is supremely important is that healthy and sick people alike find that [it is] faith in Christ which judges and redeems their earthly striving."[22]

This analysis is accurate, however, only if one limits the definition of health to the physical. It is true that there are times when sacrifice of physi-cal health for the good of someone else's health or life is necessary—heroic self-sacrifice. "Health is not an end in itself; it is significant only insofar as life itself is significant."[23] Even physical life can be a god that doctors wor-ship—the highest good. But if health is wholeness and synonymous with sal-vation, then it is the highest virtue and our goal. (This wholeness is under-stood as *beatitudo* in Thomistic terms.)

Wholeness depends on one's relationship with God and one's relationship with others (freedom from a state of sin) and on physical reconstruction (well-being). The biblical view is that physical well-being is only one aspect of health, that bodily health supplies but one part of salvation. The Hebrew word *raphâ* means "heal," "repair," "mend." "For God wounds, but God binds up; God strikes, but God's hands heal" (Job 5:18). In the Greek of the Christian Scriptures, what is often translated as *sōzō,* "to save," and secon-darily "to be saved, well," originally was more inclusive. "If I only touch his cloak, I will be made well" (Matt. 9:21). In the biblical tradition, health and salvation are integrally connected, and Jesus' title, Savior, also means healer.

John Wycliffe, Reformed biblical scholar, translated the word *soteria* as "health," not "salvation," in a number of texts since he regarded health as a state of life in which the physical and spiritual aspects of human nature are united in loving response to God. "Wholeness of life" may be the best trans-lation for both health and salvation. We have to deal with both aspects of human nature.[24]

Are health and salvation conflated? If so, is health the *summum bonum*? Or is health the goal of this life and salvation the goal of eternal life? Health and salvation are not equivalents, but related concepts. Health and salvation are both goals, but salvation includes the indispensable additional element of God's grace, which results in our faith in Jesus Christ as Sovereign and Savior. According to Reformed theology, works are the signs of salvation, but neither they nor faith is the cause or basis for it. Health, on the other hand, is not gratis nor does it necessarily result from a strong faith. It requires active responsibility on the part of the person for its fullest realization.

Health and salvation are also distinguished by the fact that complete health always includes physical well-being whereas salvation does not depend upon one's bodily condition. Salvation does not consist in being freed from disease or achieving society's definition of mental health. (Saviors and martyrs are notoriously labeled as mentally unbalanced.)[25] Not every Christian enjoys robust health. The apostle Paul suffered a "thorn" in the flesh for years (2 Cor. 12:7). Timothy apparently had various health problems (1 Tim. 5:23). Epaphroditus, a colleague of Paul, was seriously ill (Phil. 2:26–30). The Christian Scriptures do not assume that vital faith in God is accompanied by physical and mental well-being.[26]

Salvation differs from health since the wholeness of salvation is promised in the very midst of death. Christ's death was viewed as the way to salvation and the transformation of life in this world. Some claim that it is possible to experience the promise of salvation while being in poor physical health. Is the possible distinction between these two concepts that health is in this life and salvation in the next? The answer is no if we regard health as a process or goal, not a state that is achieved in this life. "Health is what we enjoy when we are on our way to that which God is preparing for us to enjoy. It is a value and a vision word. Practically speaking, health is never reached; it is an eschatological ideal. We seek health even as we enjoy it. . . . It is a vision beyond the range of possibilities or failures of medicine."[27]

Another dimension of the relationship of health and salvation is the connection between health, forgiveness, and obedience. (The converse of this will be examined when analyzing the relationship between sin and sickness.) Numerous scripture passages reflect this relationship:

God said, "If you will listen carefully to the voice of your God, and do what is right in God's sight, and give heed to God's commandments and keep all God's statutes, I will not bring upon you any of the diseases that I brought upon the Egyptians; for I am the One who heals you." (Exod. 15:26)

God sustains them on their sickbed;
    in their illness you heal all their infirmities.
As for me, I said, "O God, be gracious to me;
    heal me, for I have sinned against you." (Ps. 41:3–4)

Who forgives all your iniquity,
    who heals all your diseases. (Ps. 103:3)

Do not be wise in your own eyes;
    fear God, and turn away from evil.

It will be a healing for your flesh
and a refreshment for your body. (Prov. 3:7–8)

My child, be attentive to my words;
incline your ear to my sayings.
Do not let them escape from your sight;
keep them within your heart.
For they are life to those who find them,
and healing to all their flesh. (Prov. 4:20–22)

Do these passages suggest that righteousness guarantees good health as a sign of one's ultimate health? The answer is no. But one's relationship with God does have a profound effect on one's general well-being. Love of God and neighbor affects health, but provides no guarantee against sickness and suffering.

Sickness, Sin, and Suffering

Before proceeding with a discussion of sickness as brokenness, we need to reiterate the distinction between disease, illness, and sickness. The medical model reduces sickness to disease—an organic entity or malfunction to be attacked and cured. Illness equals the description of the various manifestations of disease. Rebelling against this reduction of illness to disease, psychiatrist Tristram Engelhardt and philosopher Christopher Boorse provide important distinctions between illness and disease. For Boorse, disease is a morally neutral term applied indifferently to organisms of all species. Illnesses are a subclass of disease and take on normative and value connotations.[28] A disease becomes an illness when (1) it is undesirable for its bearer; (2) special treatment is given; and (3) normally criticizable behavior is accepted.[29]

Engelhardt agrees with Boorse's analysis on the basis that one can have a disease without being ill and vice versa. To speak of disease is to convert an illness into a syndrome. Disease is whatever is undesirable.[30] "The concept of disease is used in accounting for physiological and psychological (or behavioral) disorders, offering generalizations concerning patterns of phenomena which we find disturbing and unpleasant."[31] It refers to a negative, that is, unwanted discontinuity or deviation in the condition of a person.[32] Engelhardt accepts both ontological and etiological concepts of disease, a multidimensional concept of disease that includes genetic, infectious, metabolic, psychological, and social elements. Medical and psychological models of disease should be complementary, not competitive, given the broad range of disease origin.[33] By these distinctions, both Boorse and Engelhardt reflect their rooting in psychiatry. In the field of mental health, nosologies, disease, disorder, and disturbances become especially important because how one defines what qualifies as a disease or illness will determine whether treatment is in order.

For some, sickness is defined as malfunctioning, hence distinguished from illness and disease. The definition of sickness as malfunctioning is the opposite of health as well-working and suggests the biblical view of sickness as brokenness. For Parsons, somatic illness is the incapacity for performance of relevant tasks, parallel to the sense in which mental illness is the incapacity for the performance of one's role. How one measures these is relative to one's "status" in society. In U.S. society, capacity is the primary focus, with activism and achievement highly valued.[34] "Disease is the aggregate of those conditions which, judged by the prevailing culture, are deemed painful, or disabling, and which, at the same time, deviate from either the statistical norm or from some idealized status."[35] The main problem with interpreting sickness as malfunctioning is that it emphasizes a part rather than the whole person.

Karl Barth, the twentieth-century Protestant theologian, works at a deeper level when he distinguishes between partial impotence to exercise our functions as humans and the impotence to be humans per se. Sickness may impair, disable, and hamper one or several of our powers without assaulting the essence or identity of what it means to be human.[36]

Sin and Sickness as Brokenness

A wholistic view of sickness is contained in the definition of sickness as brokenness. There are three ways of understanding sickness as brokenness: internal brokenness of a person; alienation from one's neighbor; and estrangement from God. Brokenness is an apt metaphor for defining sickness as the malfunction of all creation.[37] A family, a community, a nation, or even the physical world, in the instance of pollution, can be sick. Medically, reference is made to torn ligaments, ruptured blood vessels, or dislocated bones. More popularly, we refer to splitting headaches and split personalities—people "cracking up" or "going to pieces." All these expressions connote brokenness, separation, and division. Societal terms, such as fragmented communities, racial divisions, and schisms, describe this same brokenness. So sickness may manifest itself in different forms at different levels, but all sickness is derived from a brokenness that pervades every level of human existence.

Sickness as brokenness describes an ongoing state, not merely the experience of episodic events. It involves the whole person at every level of life, though at any given moment it may present itself specifically in the physical, emotional, mental, or spiritual dimension. A person may experience broken relationships or an alienation from the world. This brokenness from a theological perspective is called sin.

A similar definition of sin parallels this perspective on sickness. Sin refers to a separation from God, as well as disobedience of God and God's laws. Since both sin and sickness reflect brokenness in people's lives, how are they related? Are they identical? Does one cause the other? Does God send one as a punishment of the other?

The relationship between sin and sickness is important both theologically and existentially. Theologically, it raises a whole set of theodicy questions; existentially, it concerns both the patient and the healer. It touches at the heart of patients' questions: Why are they ill? Will they recover? Will they have any control over illness or recovery? For the healer, the possible relation between sin and sickness influences the type of treatment and care.

Dealing with these issues in abstract theological treatises rather than considering their interplay in concrete individuals and situations creates difficulties in answering these questions. Well people want to know what particular actions lead to negative consequences, and sick people desire to understand the relationship between prior life and current condition. The Bible addresses these questions in the context of various people's lives, not as homilies on the relationship between sin and sickness. Their relationship always proves to be complex and varied, at times paradoxical, and certainly not clear-cut.

The biblical perspective argues that sin and sickness interrelate, but not always in a causal way. Further, God figures in the mystery of their connectedness, but always to bring about ultimate goodness and health. Thus, the healer's job is not to draw theoretical relationships between them or insist on some transparent level of connection. If through conversations either the patient or healer recognizes a connection, or perhaps more important the absence of one, this discovery should form part of the treatment. This approach may free the patient from guilt that is inhibiting healing.

In the Hebrew and Christian Scriptures, sin and sickness are linked etymologically and in certain contexts are used interchangeably. Several different words are used for each of these terms. In Hebrew *kalah* means "to be rubbed" or "worn," "to be weak," "sick," "afflicted," "put to grief," or "exhausted." The Hebrew verb *pâtsam* is rendered "to split open," "break," "defile," or "wound." The Greek carries the same double meanings: *kakos* is translated "amiss," "diseased," "evil," "miserable"; *asthenēo,* "to be feeble," "sick," "weak"; *kamnō,* "to faint," "to be sick," "to be weary." Another word for sin in the Christian Scriptures, *hamartia* ("missing the mark"), is probably related to terms such as "abnormal" and "maladjusted." Sin and sickness have a common historical root in the form of alienation from God, self, or society.[38]

Are we saying then that "sickness" is a secular term for sin and "illness" for evil and that the secular terms have eclipsed the religious reality? Karl Menninger argued in that direction when he titled his book *Whatever Happened to Sin?* At this point one not only rejects the equation between sickness and sin, but also rejects the latter in favor of the former. The medical model labeled illness as involuntary, hence nonculpable and devoid of moral dimensions. In fact, one of the reasons that psychiatry adopted the medical model for treating mental illness was to remove it from the prison of a theology gone bad where exorcism and witchcraft were considered appropriate therapies for treating sickness. It is true, however, that the accompanying symptoms of sinfulness and sickness are similar, that is, feelings of guilt, "Why me?" and feelings of being unjustly punished, "What have I done to deserve this?" Both are undesirable states and manifestations of evil. Illness destroys in some of the same ways that sin does, but they are not identical.

The weight of the biblical material suggests that while personal sin is one's fault, sickness is not always a consequence of an individual's thoughts or actions. Because we are part of the human race, we suffer the consequences of our fallen human nature as well as experience the joys of being human. As we enjoy the assets of life—sun, rain, beauty, sleep, freedom, which we may not directly create or warrant—so we suffer the liabilities of life—epidemics, tornadoes, wars for which we may not be directly responsible.

Sin and sickness are not identical because sickness may have a nonculpable dimension that sin lacks. Only acts for which one is responsible can be termed sinful, though suffering in one person's life may result from someone else's sin. Sickness may recur through no fault of one's own, for example, as part of an epidemic, but sinfulness is always at least partly one's responsibility. Does sickness result from sin? From a Judeo-Christian perspective, there are two aspects to this question: (1) our responsibility for our sickness due to a sinful nature or acts, and (2) God's use of sickness as a punishment for sin.

In relation to the first aspect, the story of the Fall describes a spiritual break between God and humankind, which resulted in suffering and death. According to the Genesis account, suffering in all its forms is mentioned together with death as a consequence of sin. There are obvious examples of how the misuse and abuse of one's body, the aimlessness of one's life, and the mistreatment of others can cause one's illness as well as affect future generations. Furthermore, both psychological and physical ailments may be caused or exacerbated by guilt or remorse for sin. When sin has been forgiven and the burden of guilt removed, the illness often disappears.[39]

Hebrew Scriptures' View of Sickness

A number of scriptural passages attribute sickness and even death to sin or view sickness as a direct punishment from God, for example, "the devastation of that land and the afflictions with which God has afflicted it" (Deut. 29:22). To appreciate what the writers were saying about the relation of sin and sickness, we need to understand the attitudes prevalent at the time the Hebrew Scriptures were written.

Many Hebrews believed that any sickness was a sign of moral disorder within the person. A sick person was a sinner; the sickness reflected God's disfavor rather than being a symptom of an organic disorder. Hence healing was possible only by God's forgiveness. For example, King Asa suffered a severe foot disease and was criticized for consulting physicians instead of God (2 Chron. 16:12). Ill people were expected to seek the priest's forgiveness for their sins, which would lead to physical healing.

Numerous passages from the Hebrew Scriptures directly correlate sickness and God's punishment. Miriam spoke against Moses and was smitten with leprosy for seven days (Num. 12:9–15). Leprosy struck Gehazi, Elisha's servant, for his lies and greed (2 Kings 5:27). Uzziah's leprosy resulted from his arrogant pride (2 Chron. 26:19–20). Eli died because he allowed his sons to run rampant (1 Sam. 3:13; 4:17–18).

The story of Jehoram, king of Judah in the ninth century B.C.E., further illustrates the Hebrew Scriptures' point of view (2 Chron. 21). Jehoram seduced the people to idolatry and murdered his brothers and the princes. Those sins were punished by a plague on his people, family, and property, and his own sickness. Their fulfillment was carried out by the Philistines and Arabians, who conquered Judah, and his painful, slow disease for which there was no cure. Some believe the disease was a violent dysentery—an inflammation of the tissue of the large intestine that causes the overlying mucous membrane to decay and peel off and fall out, often in a tube shape, so that the intestines appear to fall from the body. We are left with no doubt that in the Chronicler's mind, Jehoram's sickness and death were a direct punishment from God for his sin.

From the Deuteronomic point of view, the arrogantly idolatrous person is liable to God's anger with sickness as a curse from God. "But if you will not obey me, and do not observe all these commandments . . . I in turn will do this to you: I will bring terror on you; consumption and fever that waste the eyes and cause life to pine away" (Lev. 26:14–16).

Not only did the prophetic and historical writers draw a causal relationship between sin and sickness, but so did the writers of the poetical books, especially the psalmist. (See, for example, Pss. 6:1–2; 38:3–7; 41:3–4; 103:3; Prov. 3:7–8.) Psalm 107 introduced the idea of sickness as the result of human sin, but God is the One who delivers us from sickness when we repent. In other words, God, not a capricious natural law, is in control of sickness and health. This view of sickness as a punishment from God discouraged the development of medical science among the pre-Dispersion Jews. Since sin caused sickness and sin must be forgiven before healing could take place, only priests practiced medicine.

However, even for the Jews the story of Job carried a warning against the oversimplified view that all sickness was the direct result of a particular person's sin. Job was a righteous man. He had everything—material riches, a fine family, a high social position, and everyone's respect. Then those goods disappeared—animals, servants, and children. Job's reaction was, "Naked I came from my mother's womb, and naked shall I return there; God gave, and God has taken away; blessed be the divine name" (Job 1:21). Yet his trials were not over. Next, open sores covered his entire body, and he went off to sit on a garbage dump. His wife deserted him, suggesting that he curse God and die. At first, his friends, seeing his great suffering, could only sit in silence. At length, their talk only added to his miseries. They accused Job of horrible sins of which he must repent in order to be forgiven by God.

After Job cried out to God for vindication, God answered that he should not question the reason for his suffering. The prose epilogue concludes that since Job remained faithful and believed in God, his possessions, children, and health were restored many times over.

Job's reaction to the events instructs us concerning the possible connection between sin and sickness. As the drama unfolded, Job passed through various emotions: numbness, uncertainty, rage, doubt, discouragement, hope, repentance, and vindication. But he never cursed God. Although he insisted on his righteousness, he did not maintain that he was sinless, only that he was not sinful enough to deserve all that he experienced. At length, when the weight of his suffering bore down with all its force, Job cursed his birth and speculated that God had put a curse on the day he was born (Job 3:2–3) and had lined up terrors against him (Job 16). As Job experienced the ravages of his disease and the isolation from his friends, he likened himself to a mourner (Job 30) and saw death as his only release (Job 6, 7). While Job stopped short of cursing God, he continually cried out to God for an explanation of the various catastrophes. He asked two things of God: relief from suffering and release from the absurdity that he could not present his case.

Job was torn between believing that God was so powerful God was unapproachable and that God would answer him directly. He realized the gulf that separated him from God and wanted an arbitrator between them: "For God is not a mortal, as I am, that I might answer God, that we should come to trial together. There is no umpire between us, who might lay his hand on us both" (Job 9:32–33). When God finally spoke, Job was overcome. He said, "Then I knew only what others had told me, but now I have seen you with my own eyes" (Job 42:5).[40] He repented in dust and ashes for trying to be equal with God, and he realized that his works were nothing in relation to the Creator of the universe.

Job's friends, on the contrary, reflected the theology of their day about the relationship of sin and sickness. Eliphaz, Bildad, and Zophar were united in their judgment of Job. They all sounded the theme that Job must repent of his sin to eliminate his suffering. They did not pay much attention to Job or the facts before them, but dealt instead in pious, irrelevant platitudes. Their initial reaction of horrified silence at the miserable sight of Job gave way to increasingly judgmental diatribes against their former friend. Rather than being a comfort to him, they seemed to be yet another trial sent by Satan. They erred chiefly in applying relative truths absolutely to every situation.

One awaits eagerly God's resolution of the conflict between Job and his friends about the connection between sickness and sin. Scripture highlights three features of God's response to Job: first, God spoke directly to Job; second, God's message offered a challenge more than an answer; and third, God's actions reflected God's love and vindication of Job.

God referred to the wonders of creation and the mystery that it presents. Job, who had been claiming wisdom, was not even there when wisdom wrought its principles in the creation of the world. God cited control of the sea, which represented restlessness and evil forces, God's creation of light and darkness, and other mysteries of the heavens and the earth of which God is the source. God reminded Job of his human limitations and the fact that he could not contest with God as an equal. The reason for Job's suffering was not really explained. Ultimately, a mystery remains. However, the story provides insights into the relation between suffering, sin, and sickness: Satan, not God, is the author of evil; God cares for people in the midst of their suffering; if sickness is not immediately healed, God gives the strength and patience to endure; God's goodness eventually triumphs.

Christian Scriptures' Perspectives on Sickness

This complexity in the relationship between sin and sickness carries forward into the Christian Scriptures. On the one hand, Jesus implied that sickness is the work of demons (Matt. 12). Both sin and sickness are regarded as works of the devil, and victory over them is a sign of God's incoming reign. When Jesus healed someone who was mentally ill, the sufferer was regarded not as a sinner but as the victim of strong satanic forces. Jesus exorcised the demon rather than called the sufferer to repent (Mark 1:21–27).

Some scholars believe that there is no distinction in the Christian Scriptures between sickness linked to sins (Luke 4:40–41), and sickness as a result of demon possession: "He cast out the spirits with a word, and cured all who were sick" (Matt. 8:16). Jesus' healing was a sign of the authentication of Christ's teaching and preaching in God's name.[41] Although Early Christianity was aware of its power to heal, healing was still a theme of prayer (2 Cor. 12:8). In response to the accusation of the Pharisees that he was allied with Satan, Jesus asked how Satan could cast out Satan, and he went on to declare, "If I cast out demons by Beelzebul, by whom do your own exorcists cast them out? Therefore they will be your judges" (Matt. 12:27).

On the other hand, after healing the man who was paralyzed, Jesus tells him to sin no more lest a worse thing befall him (Luke 5:17–26). In this story, Jesus links physical healing and the forgiveness of sins. The man's illness was readily seen by everyone; the Greek word for "paralysis," *paralutikos,* indicates a disease of some part of the nervous system, which meant he could do nothing but lie in bed. His body was disabled, but Jesus saw as well that his spirit needed to be healed, so first he forgave his sins.

Paul, reflecting the Deuteronomic point of view, appeared to correlate a person's sin and sickness in relation to the incorrect partaking of Holy Communion (1 Cor. 11:29–30). James 5 states that the prayer of faith will save the sick person, and if one has committed sins, the person will be forgiven (healed). Sickness here is regarded as a special opportunity to take stock, to examine oneself concerning the reasons for illness.

There are cases mentioned in the Christian Scriptures where sickness or even death was seen as a direct punishment from God. Ananias and Sapphira were struck dead because they lied about the purchase of property (Acts 5:1–11). Herod Agrippa I was eaten by worms because he did not give God the glory in his reign (Acts 12:23).

In the midst of these stories relating sin and sickness comes the account of the man who was born blind. This story disturbs the pat answers, just as the story of Job questioned the Hebrews' correlation of sin and sickness. The story addresses the question whether sickness is always God's will and a punishment for sin. Everyone operates with a different set of presuppositions. Jesus upsets everyone's stereotypes and restores physical sight and gives spiritual insight to one man, but is unable to restore spiritual sight to the others, that is, the Pharisees.

Jesus' disciples ask the central question, "Rabbi, who sinned, this man or his parents, that he was born blind?" (John 9:2). Jesus disrupts all their expectations by stating that neither one had sinned. Then he adds that God's power will be manifest through the man's healing. While the disciples are carrying on a theological debate and the Pharisees are worried about the observance of the Sabbath, Jesus is involved with God's main concern, to abolish suffering. After the man is healed, the Pharisees cast him out. Upon finding Jesus, he accepts Jesus as the Messiah, hence extending his healing to include spiritual wholeness.

Patristic teaching carried forward the interpretation that sin and sickness were related. For example, Cyprian, in his writing *On the Lapsed,* believed the denial of Christ brought all kinds of disasters including illness. This carries into a belief that salvation is of both the body and the spirit. Saint Ignatius, Justin Martyr, and Clement of Alexandria all referred to the union of the two in constituting what it means to be human, hence transformation in Christ will affect both of them.[42] In conclusion, however, the Scriptures and the church teach that sickness is part of the imperfect world, but there is not a necessary connection between individual sickness and sin.

6

HEALING AS MOVING TOWARD WHOLENESS

What difference does it make to our present understanding to have examined the concepts of health and sickness from the Judeo-Christian perspective? Just this. Conceiving health as wholeness expands the understanding of healing. Healing is any activity or attitude that moves one toward wholeness—a wholeness greater than the sum of its parts. It restores harmony with oneself, God, and the world; healing is akin to the Hebrew understanding of *shalom*.

AN EXPANDED VISION OF HEALTH AND HEALING

Definitions of sickness are not mere word exercises, but essential to the whole theology of healing. Morality and values do not simply impinge on medical ethics but on the whole understanding of illness and healing. Different methods challenge not only other practices of healing but also fundamental values and worldviews. The ways one defines the purpose and substance of illness say a lot about one's belief systems as well as the methods of healing that one employs.[1] What is God trying to tell us through illness? The meaning of illness is one of the most important questions we face.

By focusing almost exclusively on disease, contemporary medicine fails to offer a vision for health that would heighten expectations of healing. The resulting truncated view of healing shortchanges the patient by offering only cure and a piecemeal approach to illness, which fails to treat the whole person. Revisionists such as Cassell and Pellegrino describe wholistic illness and the physician's art of healing, but fail to move past an individualistic view of health and to provide a comprehensive understanding of the relevant parties in the enterprise of healing.

Healing may entail freedom from oppression where powerless and marginalized persons are so debilitated by their position in society that the slightest illness may overwhelm them completely. Healing also involves empowering us through knowledge. For example, in the patient self-help movement understanding and being in touch with what is happening to the body can help one overcome the feeling of helplessness that can inhibit healing. Healing naturally includes curing of physical illness and restoring of mental, emotional, and spiritual health.

As psychology has given new insights about healing to physical medicine, so spiritual healing may introduce new methods to both. As far back as the ante-Nicene church, important insights into spiritual healing were shared when the saints' faith and prayer overcame material circumstances.[2] One recognizes the interdependence of the physical, the mental, and the spiritual. The boundary between healing classified as miraculous or inexplicable and healing in conformity with laws of nature is constantly changing.[3]

Broadened definitions of healing appear to legitimize any activity that moves toward wholeness. One fears this may open the way to all sorts of exotic practices. How does one avoid the *extremes* of the holistic health movement? How can one license a wider group of healers and regulate the procedures they practice? Skepticism is justified. As Santayana expressed it, "Skepticism is the chastity of the mind." Further, some practices fall in a middle ground between traditional medicine and holistic techniques such as therapeutic touch (TT). TT was introduced into the nursing profession in the early seventies by Delores Krieger, and now some conservatively estimated fifteen thousand nurses use it, including medical centers such as Columbia University. Under controlled laboratory conditions distinct biological changes have been noted. The practitioner needs to be "centered" (a state of relaxation where all personal considerations are put aside). TT may not involve literal touching, but is a way of experiencing or feeling the electromagnetic energy field of another person.[4] One must use both theological and scientific rigor in assessing the use of this and other avant-garde resources for healing.

A broader definition of healing may also promise more than it can deliver. It may feed into the American aspiration for perfection, a utopianism that eventually disappoints. Realism argues for the tempering of expectations. Once tempered, the patient may come to appreciate that while complete healing may not be possible, some healing is always available—deterrents to health are removed. "The healed man . . . is a man in whom the obstacles to the development of his true nature have been eliminated."[5] What are the obstacles that need to be eliminated, or put positively, what factors contribute to health? Consider the following: genetic (what one has received through one's parents); physiological (how one's body has developed); sociological (the natural and human environment); economic (class, income); lifestyle (job, marital status, diet, exercise); philosophical/theological (value system and religious beliefs); and psychological (one's self-esteem and integration of personality).

Verifiable data in the last several decades about the importance of most of these factors as contributing to health have led to their general acceptance. However, heretofore, little statistical evidence was available concerning religion and its contribution to total health.

Various means may be used by the patient herself, family, friends, church members, and traditional health care professionals. These include physical methods such as diet, adequate sleep, exercise, clean water, and adequate housing; medical means such as surgery, drugs, medical procedures, and treatments; emotional factors such as affection, touch, compassion, presence of friends and family, support groups and self-help groups, and the offering of hope; spiritual resources such as offering hope, prayer and worship, and faith of friends and the patient; psychological means such as counseling, therapy, and imaging. (The means open to the church in her health ministry will be discussed in depth in my companion volume.) As one embraces a more wholistic vision of healing, all the resources that God has made available are means of God's healing grace. No one owns or controls the process of healing. However, there are a number of ways of getting germs and injuries out of the way of healing—ways to redirect the healing process—but not how to cause it. Healing is a God-given process with which one can only cooperate.

Trevor Nash, president of Guild of Health in the United Kingdom, says healing is to set men, women, and children free to be able to begin to love God, their neighbor, and themselves, and to know the immensity of God's love for them. Morris Maddocks has defined Christian healing as Jesus Christ meeting us at the point of our need.[6] Wholeness means the whole of life, including illness, disability, old age, and death. It is not some perfect ideal, but life as one knows it changed into a channel for God. It is the quality of life lived within the circumstances of wellness or sickness. Wholeness in this life does not mean perfection, flawlessness, success, or completion. Complete fulfillment will come only through dying. Growing into wholeness will be determined by what one makes of one's impairments. As we grow into a right relationship with God, we are indeed beginning to be made whole. Healing is not about being restored to a state in the past or even about being restored to full function. Healing is concerned with new growth, new understanding, a new development in the future, even including death.[7]

The Communal Dimensions of Healing

Healing from a Judeo-Christian perspective is concerned not only with individual health but also with the well-being of neighbor, community, and world. Furthermore, if others are not whole, one cannot be in complete health. This is tied to the earlier discussion that a Christian's concern should be for others' health.

However, healing in contemporary society operates from a wholly different perspective. It draws on an individualistic, interventionist model of eradicating disease, which reflects itself in both contemporary medicine and religion—a deliverance model. The patient has a physical or spiritual problem, then goes to the doctor or pastor to have it removed. In the medical model, health becomes an achievement of the doctor, not the patient. Some modifications of this model include the needs of the whole person—body, mind, and soul—but seldom the communal dimension of healing. This individualistic approach to healing produces a concept of the "good," that is, health, salvation, riches, to be achieved by extracting the "bad," that is, disease, sin, poverty. Therefore, the surgeon preeminently symbolizes the healer as he extracts a localizable problem with a knife, as a priest removes sin by absolution.

Robert Lambourne, a British psychiatrist and pastoral theologian who died several decades ago, has suggested some interesting interactions between Christian theology and medicine that encouraged this individualistic view toward healing.[8] The structures and organizations formed by priests and doctors resemble one another—a church building–centered religion and a hospital-centered medicine—both obsessed with extracting defects from individuals. The sinner (sick person) must come out of the environment (home) to be saved (healed) by the professional priest (doctor) in a church building (hospital) by a technical process that the professional alone defines and administers. The church departed from its origins in the corporate experience of the deliverance from sins and the promise of a new life in Holy Communion, a sacrament once performed in the home by lay leaders, using ordinary elements.

The biblical perspective emphasizes the communal dimension of healing—caring for people who are ill in their milieu. The Hebrew Scriptures are essentially about a community. The Genesis account of creation emphasizes the importance of human beings living in relationship: "It is not good that the man should be alone; I will make him a helper as his partner" (Gen. 2:18). The Hebraic concept of corporate personality blurs the boundaries between an individual and those to whom one relates. One represents the many—the man, his household; the patriarch, his tribe; the king, his people; the priest on Yom Kippur, the whole people; and finally the Suffering Servant, the whole of humankind.[9] Jesus Christ as the Suffering Servant, the Human One, represents all people—as in Adam all people die, so in Christ all will live (Rom. 5). Hence, an individual's health and personal salvation are intertwined with those of the community.

Response to this communal dimension of healing is not simply creating an interdisciplinary team of healers in the fashion of the Wholistic Health Care Centers, Inc. While the movement constitutes an important recognition of the multifaceted nature of healing, it offers little critique of the community or society, which frequently causes the individual's illness and itself stands in need of healing. Instead, we must recognize our responsibility for others' health. Lacking wholeness, one person disturbs the wholeness of others. Carrying one another's burdens moves us toward wholeness. Judeo-Christian theology provides a perspective for moving away from a self-centered approach to health or a narrow view of healing.

BIBLICAL WORDS RELATED TO HEALING

Examining the variety of words in the Christian Scriptures for healing is instructive in understanding the comprehensive nature of healing from the biblical perspective. They point to its broad meaning. *In Community, Church, and Healing,* Lambourne refers to the various words used to describe the healing miracles, *therapeuō, iaomai, katharizō, apokathistēmi,* and *sōzō,* that link healing and saving. This shows the connection between them, but it is not to be thought of as a mathematical ratio.[10]

We will now look more closely at the broad set of words connected to our definitions of healing. In secular Greek and in the intertestamental period *therapeuō* meant "to be serviceable," "to serve for the good of those involved." There was only a small amount of evidence to show it was used of healing. However, in the Christian Scriptures it was used a great deal in the sense of healing, in the work of Jesus (for example, Matt. 4:23; 9:35; Mark 3:10; Luke 5:15; 6:18; 7:21; 9:11), and in the commission to the disciples to do likewise (Luke 10:9). The word literally means "to attend to" or "to tend." The *therapon* were servants, attendants, or ministers. The root of the word "therapeutic" literally means the "act of attending"; later it referred to the "act of healing." In the Septuagint, for example, Numbers 12:7, it was the word chosen to translate "servant" and referred to Moses' attendants. There also was a first-century sect of Jewish mystics residing in Egypt, who were described in Philo's *Concerning the Contemplative Life.* They were similar to the Essenes, who lived a life of extreme asceticism.[11]

The Greek verb *iaomai,* meaning "to cure" or "heal," is a medical term in classical Greek and was used primarily by Luke. It also had a moral connotation, but Luke used it in place of *therapeuō* in the commission of the Twelve (Luke 9:2; Matt. 10:8). All the Synoptic Gospels use it for the work of Jesus. Although it directly relates to healing, as in its secular use, it also carries the sense of Jesus' wider ministry, for example, in being restored spiritually from a state of sin (Matt. 13:15).

The Greek verb *katharizō* carries the meaning of "to cleanse" and "purify" the internal self. For example, it is found in Acts 15:9, "And in cleansing their hearts . . . made no distinction," and in Titus 2:14, "Purify for himself a people of his own who are zealous for good deeds." The concept of purification ties to one's understanding of spiritual health where the inner nature and the outer nature are made whole.

The Greek verb *egeirō* in its secular meaning was "to awaken" from sleep. In the Gospels it was used to mean "healing of the sick" in the sense of "he came and took her by the hand and lifted her up," "he touched her hand . . . and she got up," and "stand up, take your bed and go to your home" (Mark 1:31; Matt. 8:15; 9:6). In addition, *egeirō* was used to convey the idea of resurrection in both the physical sense and the spiritual sense.

The Greek verb *apokathistēmi* has the sense of "to restore" to an earlier condition. This restoration could be of anything—a borrowed article, a building, or a political state—and was used of the future restoration of Israel. As well, it referred to healing a person (Mark 3:5; 8:25).

Another term related to this broader understanding of healing is *metanoia* (change of mind, repentance), which is a prerequisite for forgiveness and connotes restoration to the fellowship of believers. Repentance and forgiveness of sins are linked, for example, in Jesus' last words to his disciples (Luke 24:47). Even more interesting is the movement in 2 Corinthians 7:9–11 from godly grief to repentance to salvation. So repentance leads to healing. "Reconciliation," *katallage,* describes the changed relationship between God and humankind through Christ and then between people. As 2 Corinthians 5:16–19 points out, we become a new creation because we are reconciled. Becoming new affects body, mind, and spirit—an expanded understanding of healing that is a gift from God (Rom. 5:11).

The Greek verb *hugiainō* means to be "healthy," but also carries the sense of "soundness" or "wholeness." Its root is taken from the name Hygeia, the Greek goddess of health, and is the origin of the English word "hygiene," as discussed in chapter 3. It is used by Luke 5:31, John 3:2, and 3 John 2 ("Beloved, I pray that all may go well with you and that you may be in good health, just as it is well with your soul").

The Greek verb *sōzō* is the most important word in the Christian Scriptures that clarifies the meaning of healing. The similarities between healing and saving are reflected in the definition of sickness as a crisis and healing as a positive response to that crisis. A crisis is a symptom of a cosmic disorder, displaced in a local failure. Healing is a "satisfactory response to a crisis, made by a group of people, both individually and corporately."[12]

If healing is any activity that moves us toward wholeness, what is the difference from a theological perspective between healing and saving? This question was discussed as well in the section about salvation and health. First, they are closely related since both have their source in God. Their closeness is particularly evident when healing becomes an occasion for recognizing God's saving care. Such was the case with the man who had leprosy and returned to thank Jesus for the healing he had experienced.[13] Second, in the biblical Greek and Hebrew the same word *sōzō* in Greek and in Hebrew means both "save" and "heal." Also it carries the meaning to "preserve" or "keep from harm," "save" (from death) or "rescue." The latter meaning is also understood in classical Greek.[14] Christ came to save those who were lost, and that was accomplished by overcoming death; hence it is not surprising that the word with its double entendre was often used. The verb is found more than one hundred times in the Gospels. It was used in the sense of being snatched from peril or threat as reflected in the stories of danger aboard ship (Matt. 8:25), or relating to the cross (Matt. 27:49; Mark 15:30–31). It also means being saved from spiritual danger, as individuals (Mark 10:26; John 5:34; 10:9) and the world as a whole (John 3:17; 12:47).

Sōzō also had the sense in secular Greek of being cured and staying in good health. It is used repeatedly in the Gospels relating to healing, always in the Synoptics, and usually in the phrase "your faith has . . . you." Of the English translations only Tyndale has held on to the positive sense of healing—Jesus bringing wholeness rather than just saving from sin. Donald Coggan notes Tyndale's translation of Luke 19:9 ("this day health has come to thy house") and says he made luminous the deep interest of Christ, for true health is impossible apart from Christ.[15] To see the link between salvation and healing is to recognize the full sense of wholeness.

Third, heal and save are joined by the act of forgiveness when the obstacles to health and salvation are removed by this freeing act. Myung-Soo Lee, a Korean theologian, defines healing as salvation of the human or of the society.[16] These are both types of healing that embody the realm of God on earth.

HEALING AS RESOLVING A CRISIS

Moving from the biblical images of healing, another aspect of healing is that of resolving a crisis. The definition of sickness as crisis moves the activity exclusively from the medical world and draws on any discipline and profession that assists people in solving a crisis. This becomes an opportunity for individual growth. Responding positively to crises becomes a signpost of moving toward wholeness. Lambourne illustrates the complexity of healing by the following example. A sick child, after a long illness, is cured, but the parents divorce; in another situation, the child dies, but the parents mend a previously broken marriage. How do we define healing in these cases? Lambourne uses no medical terms in his definition because he widens the circle of healers to include the priest, social worker, physician, and psychiatrist. This definition does not refer to one sick person but includes everyone who, by choice or accident, is involved in the crisis.

The use of the word "crisis" unifies the ministry of curing and the ministry to the dying. It makes possible one medical philosophy for the curable and the dying, which is needed to confront the anxiety that terminal illness can create. Crisis, in Lambourne's vocabulary, is seen as a positive state that can lead to a higher quality of life. One does not just survive crises but grows through them; one does not return to a previous state but moves upward. Crisis is an opportunity that may be grasped or lost.[17] The use of the term "satisfactory response" may include prayer, penicillin, clean water, sanitation, sacrament, and surgery. In terms of response, each crisis that presents itself may have more than one dimension.

Based on this definition, whoever desires healing is sick; whoever feels no need for healing is well. The need for healing does not depend on manifesting a clinically or statistically verifiable disease. Someone may have a health problem, but not a clinical medical problem. Furthermore, health may be maintained or regained in the absence of clinical medical intervention, for example, improved living conditions, nutrition, sanitation, education, and so forth.[18] This definition, however, may confuse the results of sickness, that is, the crisis, with the state of illness itself.

SUFFERING AND HEALING

Continuing to explore the various definitions and means of healing, one wonders what happens when healing does not occur? William Strawson suggests that this leads us to consider both the nature and the activity of God, that is, what is God like, and what is God doing in healing?[19] At the heart of a Christian theology of healing is the problem of pain, suffering, and death. In this section, however, we will focus not on the theodicy question, but on how Christians regard the relationship between suffering and healing.

The importance of this subject is to contrast how suffering is treated by the medical model and how it might be treated in a reconstructionist view of health, healing, and healers. In the former, suffering is outside the primary enterprise. In the latter, suffering can be a key ingredient in the process. By examining the origin, nature, reality, and effects of suffering, we are better able to confront and not deny it. The struggle to understand suffering is part of the healing process.

David Smith, a philosopher and ethicist, makes a significant distinction between pain and suffering. Pain is mainly a physical sensation. While suffering can be produced by intense pain, it is much more, that is, "suffering is associated with a disruption in the coherence and order that I perceive in the world."[20]

The Reality of Suffering

Suffering forms part of a theology of healing. Suffering is a universal, inexplicable mystery. Suffering may be caused by shame in a family, loss of job, poor health, bad lifestyle choices, a pessimistic worldview, permanent disability, loneliness, rejection, broken relationships and marriages, physical pain, or the tragic loss of a loved one. All these experiences produce suffering. Smith's suggestion that genuine suffering is something that appears purposeless is an important observation, for in genuine suffering one's whole being stands on the precipice of dissolution.[21] Suffering threatens our whole sense of self.

Suffering inevitably raises the question of why bad things happen to good people, and Harold S. Kushner's popular book *When Bad Things Happen to Good People* addressed that topic. Pierre Wolf, the Jesuit priest who counsels people recovering from tragedies, suggests that suffering occurs when winter enters one's life. Suffering is an anguish, a threat to who one is, to composure, to identity.[22]

This same theme is powerfully developed by Martin Marty, Evangelical Lutheran Church of America clergy and theologian par excellence, in *A Cry of Absence*. No one can escape the winter of the heart, and acknowledging that reality is at the core of the believer's struggle.[23] Summer-style believers seem to shun the doubter and offer a Christianity of cool comfort. Winter Christians often find themselves alongside the atheists living on the edges of doubt but still struggling to include a yes to God.[24] Marty draws heavily on Karl Rahner, the great twentieth-century German scholar, agreeing with him that we need not eliminate a summer Christianity, but neither should it be allowed to have the only voice.[25]

A reconstructionist's view might respond to suffering not by viewing it as external to the healing process, as in the medical model, but by incorporating it into the center of the enterprise. In the introduction to her book *Hallelujah Anyhow*, Diedra Kriewald says, "We should name the pain; enter into the suffering; let go; witness to the power of God."[26]

Although modern medicine has been quite successful in curing an incredible range of illnesses, it does not have an adequate perspective to address the problem of suffering. When medical practitioners do address suffering, they are moving beyond the strict bounds of their discipline, often with good motives and with good effects. What is needed, however, is a view of suffering that makes it a central part of the human experience and treats it in an integrated, not an ad hoc, fashion. The problem this creates, of course, is that suffering does not lend itself to a clear, systematic, and integrated treatment.

The Origin and Nature of Suffering

Underlying our previous discussion of the relation of sin and sickness was the question of suffering. Is suffering sent, permitted, or used by God? Probably the most that can be said at this point is that suffering is an opportunity, an opportunity that arises out of the potentially cataclysmic nature of suffering.

Suffering for Christ's sake is a major theme in the Christian Scriptures, for example, 1 Peter 3:17; 4:13. Paul distinguished between suffering for the sake of the gospel and "evil" from which God will rescue us (2 Tim. 4:5, 18). Distinguishing between sickness and suffering is important. Suffering may be a result of one's actions or a result of the evil world in which one lives. Suffering may be an occasion for spiritual growth, but not always. If one remains faithful to God, God may bring good out of suffering.

Popular views to the contrary (see, especially, Kushner, *When Bad Things Happen to Good People*), suffering is not a sign of God's absence from the world. However, it challenges us to entertain the notion that God is the author of evil. (Smith asserts that God's ultimate responsibility for evil is admitted up front, but that does not discredit God.) Any other conclusion may eliminate God from history and result in a deist theology. As the story of Job reflected, suffering is a mystery, but God's goodness ultimately triumphs.[27] Nevertheless, as Marty warns us, we cannot rush too quickly to that triumph; we may experience a January thaw—a brief reprise—but still be in the valley of the shadow.[28]

Suffering may be a natural consequence of a fallen world, but that does not mean God sends it as a deliberate punishment. Suffering may originate from things over which we have no control, such as earthquakes, wars, epidemics, or drunk drivers, or it may be global in nature, such as oppression, hunger, and powerlessness. God does not will everything that happens, but God wills something in everything that happens.[29] Good may come out of suffering, but that does not justify it. The good news of the gospel is not just good views but the transformation that a life in Christ may bring; sharing suffering with Christ may redeem it. Christ himself experienced the ultimate pain of unjustified suffering, freeing us ultimately.

Suffering may be a spiritual response to a physical pain. Suffering may be subtle and slow like growing old. It may stem from a feeling of emptiness that results from the loss of loved ones by separation or death or destruction of a relationship. It may result from sickness, pain, or fear of death. Fear of death permeates all experiences of suffering, which at its heart reflects humanity's vulnerability and creatureliness.

In Christian theology, suffering for righteousness' sake, persecution for one's beliefs, sanctifies suffering by giving it a purpose. Paul referred to this experience in Romans 8:18: "I consider that the sufferings of this present time are not worth comparing with the glory about to be revealed to us."

Suffering may dismantle well-established beliefs. One may say, "I don't understand anything about God anymore, why God allowed this, or whether God can do anything about it." Ultimately, the Scriptures and Christ's life, as well as the lives of the saints, leave the questions of the why of suffering unresolved. We are left most often with the absence of God[30] or, as Helmut Thielicke described it in his book of the same title, "the silence of God."

Taken together, these characteristics may provide a clue about how suffering can be incorporated into a reconstructionist's view of health, healing, and healers. One of the most important dimensions of suffering for Christians is the recognition that God is with us in our suffering. This affirmation, by its very nature, places suffering in the realm of the transcendent. It forces us to view events not in their immediate context but in the context of God and the evolution of the universe. Even when the winter seems to go on too long, there are small signs of God's presence.

In many respects, this may not be terribly helpful to the one who asks, "Why me?" or "Why is there suffering at all?" These are the fundamental questions of theodicy to deflect, not to resolve. Deflecting them is achieved by accepting the reality of "evil" and suffering and by searching for their possible implications for the healing enterprise. The place to start is the suffering of Christ; suffering was at its greatest when it was least deserved. Thus, God's greatest work may take place on the road through suffering.

Suffering and physical pain are not always synonymous. The false dichotomy between mind and body has inhibited our ability to ease suffering. To address the question of suffering, we need an understanding of humankind in its entirety. Most generally, suffering can be defined as the state of severe distress associated with events that threaten the intactness of the person.[31] The loss of hope may intensify this distress. Suffering is at the heart of a Christian understanding of healing. Healing is akin to the unleashing of the explosive force inherent in the act of creation. It is a power in nature that can even use suffering for ultimate good and incorporates setbacks into the evolutionary process.[32]

In the ante-Nicene literature three sources of suffering are described. First, the evil source is from sin and the fall of humankind. Second, the natural source is the law of the natural order, where God is ultimately but not immediately responsible. Third, God is the source when suffering is used for educational and redemptive purposes.[33] The latter is certainly the theme of Hebrews 2, especially verse 10 ("it was fitting that God . . . should make the pioneer of their salvation perfect through sufferings"). The redemptive path of suffering or the vocation of suffering is described in Philippians 1:12 ff. and 1 Peter 4:1–2.

The ante-Nicene fathers, in discussing the evil sources of sin, referenced numerous biblical passages. Christ spoke of "a daughter of Abraham whom Satan bound" (Luke 13:16) and of an unclean spirit (Mark 5:8). In working out the consequences of sin Jesus referred to the fall of Jerusalem and the collapse of the tower in Siloam (Luke 13:1–5). Sufferings caused by conflict with evil are most notably seen in Christ's life (Eph. 6:12).

The early theologians made frequent reference to evil as the source of suffering. Justin Martyr spoke of God entrusting our care to angels who protect us from demons. Tertullian referred to both kinds of evil, evils of sin and ontological evil. Origen argued that God did not produce evil even though God can bring good out it. If there is no sin, there is no suffering, according to Tertullian. Clement of Alexandria saw it as a rod of discipline used by Christ. God's power is required for suffering to have any efficacy.

According to Strawson, there are several ways of looking at suffering, not all of which are compatible: suffering is not real; it exists but is not evil because good comes out of it; it is inevitable and a natural part of the world based on human freedom.[34] At a minimum, however, one can agree that suffering is part of the lot of being human. The way one faces suffering determines to a great extent the kind of person one is. Miguel de Unamuno in his classic on suffering defined it as the substance of life and the root of personality that make us persons.[35]

Responding to Suffering

Given the above understanding of the many facets of suffering, one may now examine how the response to suffering can become a key ingredient in the reconstructionist's view of health, healing, and healers. Because of the belief that God participates in all human suffering, one may thus view suffering as an opportunity. It is an opportunity that goes well beyond the restoration of the status quo, that is, well-working.

The enigma one faces in thinking about this is that there is no clear answer to the questions, Opportunity for what? and How does this relate to healing? The answers to both questions will reside in one's understanding of the purpose and meaning of existence. Healing, in this context, will refer to the realignment of oneself on the path God intended.

Suffering, in this context, becomes the catalyst to spiritual development, for example, as Paul suggested in Romans 5 or the psalmist in Psalm 66:10 where God tests us. Suffering may bring one closer to God (Ps. 119:67). Suffering may be redemptive, as in the Suffering Servant.

The great "men and women of faith" are those who have redeemed their sufferings, have overcome adversity, have clung to hope in the midst of overwhelming odds. How we face suffering says more about us than anything else.

A key principle of the reconstructionist's view of health, healing, and healers is that suffering should be confronted. When one encounters suffering, the goal is not simply to relieve it or minimize it (as one might do through the administration of drugs to reduce the mental or physical pain that may be at the heart of the suffering). The goal is to incorporate all that has happened (or as much as is practically possible) and establish a new synthesis for the sufferer, a new and more authentic synthesis that redefines identity and how God speaks through suffering.

Peter Speck, Anglican hospital chaplain to the Royal Free Hospital, London, recounted a powerful story about facing suffering. It involved the parents of a teenage girl who had been hit by a truck while riding her new moped. The chaplain was with the father in the waiting room of the hospital as the girl hung between life and death, with severe brain damage and multiple injuries. The father became more and more agitated, asserting "God owes me a life" and demanding that the chaplain perform a miracle at that moment to save his daughter. As he yelled and screamed at the chaplain, he got down on the floor, and the chaplain knelt beside him. Finally, the story slowly emerged that the father had bought his daughter the moped and showed her how to ride it; she then set off for her first ride. The end of the road was slippery, and she skidded into the path of a truck rounding the corner. His anger at God was really anger at himself and guilt. His suffering was not only his feelings about his dying daughter but also his belief that the tragedy was his fault. The chaplain, now understanding the situation, was able to help him through his grief and assuage his guilt. Shortly afterward the daughter died, and the parents were able to accept her death and asked the chaplain for further counseling.[36]

The obvious point of the story is that the suffering had to be confronted. One does not know its long-term outcome, but the immediate results were critical. The chaplain perceived an opportunity for healing and joined with the parents in the exploration of their suffering. It seems almost certain that without the chaplain's intervention, the future lives of the parents would have been radically worsened. Whether the parents experienced spiritual development from the situation is unclear. It seems likely that extensive long-term support would be necessary. Notwithstanding, the parents could easily have been abandoned by the traditional approach to suffering.

Admittedly, the term "spiritual development" needs to be refined significantly before it can be used in this context, but the biblical tradition provides some insights. In Romans 5, Paul alluded to three stages of spiritual development through suffering: endurance, character, and hope. First, we develop endurance, as some translations render this word. As we grow older we learn that anxiety does little good; everything cannot be done yesterday. Endurance is not merely passive but an attitude of acceptance and perseverance. Endurance manifests the spirit of overcoming the world, but this does not mean that one can avoid being depressed. "We are afflicted in every way, but not crushed; perplexed, but not driven to despair; persecuted, but not forsaken; struck down, but not destroyed" (2 Cor. 4:8–9). In the depths of despair if we find God there, then there is nothing to fear.

Hence, the basis of endurance is hope. Hope is actively awaiting that moment when it can spring into action; this is not passive resignation, but determination to stick with a vision. And once one has endurance, it will produce character. Patience then produces character and character produces hope.

The word "produces" is used here to describe the process of metal passing through fire so that every impurity is removed—this is the meaning of sterling, as in sterling silver. Through the tribulation of sudden illness, we are thrust back on the essentials in life; family and friends become more important than job or money. One of Kierkegaard's major contributions was to challenge our preoccupation with the trivial and our failure to grasp the essential.[37] Because suffering throws the whole of human existence into turmoil, it becomes the opportunity to perceive correctly, perhaps for the first time, the essentials of life.

The challenge as Christians is to pass triumphantly through suffering so that we are stronger, purer, better, and nearer to God. Kierkegaard wrote, "We learn truth in proportion to our suffering." That was what Paul was saying: "Not that I am referring to being in need; for I have learned to be content with whatever I have" (Phil. 4:11). A certain exhilaration comes in knowing that we can live with crises, sickness, or pain. However, we must admit that we do not, in fact, always live through it. Sometimes the sufferings of life overwhelm.

Part of developing character is integrating disappointments into the whole life. Along with the pain one gains insights. Augustine defined virtue "as that which God works in us, without us." When one is open to God's grace, God refines the dross of experience into pure silver. Grace carries hope in her arms and bestows it as a gift in the midst of human despair. There is also at work the mystery of the dialectic—two opposite forces producing a synthesis. From the ruins of lives God builds bridgeways and walkways.

Furthermore, years of struggle and disappointment can deepen resolve and insight. Paul's thorn in the flesh occasioned him to write to the Corinthians, "We were so utterly, unbearably crushed that we despaired of life itself" (2 Cor. 1:8). But he did not completely despair: "Even though our outer nature is wasting away, our inner nature is being renewed day by day" (2 Cor. 4:16). The sense of hope in the midst of suffering is well reflected in the words of Saint Francis de Sales:

Do not look forward to the changes and chances of this life in fear; rather look to them with full hope that, as they arise, God, whose you are, will deliver you out of them. He is our keeper. He has kept you hitherto. Do you but hold fast to his dear hand, and he will lead

you safely through all things; and when you cannot stand, he will
bear you in his arms. Do not dread what may happen tomorrow. Our
Father will either shield you from suffering, or he will give you the
strength to bear it.[38]

The Christian faith proclaims that sin and sickness do not have the final
word. God's goodness and plan for this world and individuals will ultimately
prevail. Christ's life of service and sacrifice testifies how the symbols of hope
and healing are conveyed in the midst of suffering. Jesus, as the Suffering
Servant, identifies with those who are suffering.

The 1930 Lambeth Conference Committee Report drew an analogy
between temptation and sickness. We should pray for deliverance from the
evil of temptation. In the same way, we should struggle against suffering, but
sometimes the will of God dictates that we accept it. Other distinctions exist
between pain and disease. Pain may be instructive, but disease should always
be eradicated. Perhaps more helpful is the observation of Jim Wilson of the
Guild of Health that there are two types of suffering: suffering that comes
from a disease stemming from evil; and suffering that results from opposing
evil and its manifestations. The Christian is called to resist the first and
embrace the second.[39]

Christianity is not a means of escape from suffering, but a way of bringing healing through suffering. Christ's suffering on the cross is not a solution
to the problem of suffering, but a way to use it and thereby transcend it. An
important part of ministry is to support those who have tried to overcome
illness in everyday life and, when they are unsuccessful, to help them draw
closer to God.

Many passages support the idea of God's using suffering for spiritual development, for example, Paul's thorn in the flesh (2 Cor. 12:7–10). The answer
to the prayer for the removal of a thorn was not its extraction but its transformation. Paul recognized the value of suffering in the hands of God. It is a
way of correction, a means of purging from sin and strengthening of the good
in humans, and it sets our eyes on what is eternal. Paul did not view God as
the source of suffering; he saw suffering as an instrument of God's will.

In summary, the Christian faith seeks to validate suffering by giving a sense
of purpose and direction to life, a feeling of being cherished and loved, and a
conviction of a loving God whose gift is eternal life. Now, having said this, one
needs to be clear how this view of suffering provides a contrast to the medical
model and the reconstructionist's view of health, healing, and healers.

The difference, as indicated, is mainly one of perspective. In the case of
the girl who died in the moped accident, one would desire, above all, the
availability of technology that could have restored the girl's life to the
promise that it had hours before. The reconstructionist's view, however, tries

to place both the reality of the events themselves and the possibilities that they produce in a larger perspective.

The reconstructionist's view would use suffering as an opportunity for spiritual development. How this might take place will be developed later in the discussion of the differing roles of healers. The cornerstone of that process is the belief that God shares with us in our suffering and does so for God's ultimate ends. This conviction, however, may only faintly be seen, and as Marty so searingly states, even the psalmists seem most often to be left with a sense of abandonment by God with only fleeting glimpses of God's presence that breaks through in outbursts of joy.[40]

In discussing suffering, a different vision of healing has emerged in which all of the realities of sickness and ill health are recognized. As the broader definitions of health and sickness provide the foundation for a new theology of health care, the expanded concept of healing reflects a wholistic approach to our movement toward wholeness. Suffering may become a part of healing, but it remains a mystery as well. A theological perspective offers important additional dimensions to healing, but it also raises some knotty problems that are discussed in the next chapter concerning the relationship of faith and healing.

7

THE RELATIONSHIP
BETWEEN FAITH AND HEALING

Christ's healing is indicative of how God brings healing and what it means. It also raises the central question of the relationship between faith and healing. Jesus' ministry flowed directly from his compassion; his healing, caring, and teaching ministry were all interrelated. He was also engaged in spiritual warfare on a cosmic level. People in sickness and moral crisis need compassion, not judgment, in the struggle against forces they little understand.[1] Christ's presence is needed when we are overwhelmed by illness. It is not only physical illness but the sense of losing one's self-identity, of no longer being in control, of feeling completely overwhelmed by surrounding events.

JESUS' HEALING MINISTRY

The Christian Scriptures record forty healing miracles in a variety of circumstances; they represent about one-eighth of the descriptions of Jesus' life. First, Christ healed all kinds of diseases and conditions, including fevers, deafness, blindness, leprosy, dropsy, arthritis, paralysis, demonic possession, lameness, and epilepsy. Second, Jesus used a variety of healing methods: medical elements (for example, spittle, clay), physical contact, a word of command or confirmation. He responded to specific requests or healed simply out of compassion. Unlike so many self-appointed faith healers who develop certain rituals and incantations, Jesus was never bound by a methodology. Third, the results of Jesus' healing miracles were spectacular. Disabled people walked; blind people saw; demon-possessed people became coherent; dead people were raised—all ages felt his healing touch.

Proclaiming Release
From the outset of his ministry, Jesus Christ emphasized the integral connection between health and salvation. He came to heal broken relationships

as well as broken spirits, broken bodies as well as broken hearts. Initiating his ministry with the reading from Isaiah 61, Jesus indicated he would be the Servant-Messiah, both the Savior and the Healer. The passage from Isaiah quoted by Jesus (Luke 4:18) hints at the real nature of health. Health may be defined as freedom ("release to the captives") and physical well-being ("recovery of sight"). However, after he preached in the synagogue of healing and saving, the crowd tried to kill him.

In Luke's view, the remarkable initiation of Christ's ministry at Nazareth established God's rule. Following Lambourne's perspective, these were the sociopolitical realities of the realm of God breaking in, and they had primary significance for communities rather than individuals. However, Lambourne goes on to suggest that the healed person for Jesus was a representative of the community. He may go too far when he attributes Jesus' healing not to compassion for the sick person, but to a generic concern about sickness. Christ's works of healing were not purely instrumental but integral to his whole purpose of redemption.[2] Healings illustrated Christ's power, which some claim was true as well of the kings of England in Stuart times whose divine right was authenticated by their power to heal.[3] Jesus fulfilled the Hebrew Scriptures' promises of a realm characterized by health and wholeness. (See the stories of Elijah [1 Kings 17] and Elisha [2 Kings 5].) Jesus regarded disease and death as the activities of Satan and in opposition to God's reign. He stressed God's concern for the Gentiles and the universal significance of the gospel of healing.

Healing at Capernaum

Jesus had both indignation and compassion toward illness and sick people. The healing acts of Jesus sprang from mercy and love. The love of God was made manifest. There was no payment received: "You received without payment, give without payment" (Matt. 10:8). Jesus left Nazareth when he recognized the pointlessness of working against the unresponsive people of that town, and he returned to Capernaum, where he had previously performed miracles.

At Capernaum, his first act of healing restored the mind of a man possessed by demons. The Jews recognized demons as part of the kingdom of evil over which God must eventually triumph. This power of Jesus deeply impressed the crowd and certainly established his authority. Jesus' attitude toward healing was one of courage. He created a new center of consciousness from which the evil powers of sickness could be seen. Even the demons recognized him as "the Holy One of God." His authority came from both his words and his actions. Next, Jesus went to Simon's house, where he found Simon's mother-in-law fever-ridden. Jesus "rebuked the fever" (Luke 4:39), healed her, and enabled her immediately to resume her household duties. The healing of the demon-possessed man and the healing of Simon's mother-in-law were apparently just two of the healings that Christ did that day as Servant-Messiah, the Savior and the Healer. The miraculous nature of Jesus' healings established his messianic claims. It is instructive to look briefly at several of Christ's healing miracles to appreciate his healing power.

JESUS' HEALING MIRACLES

Your Faith Has Made You Whole

In Luke 8:41–56, two healing miracles are interwoven. The crowds who followed Jesus were increasing in size as news of his great power spread. He was just returning to Capernaum after curing a man possessed by demons. The two sufferers whom he met in the multitude were from completely different social classes but alike in need. One was Jairus, a prominent man in the community, "ruler of the synagogue," whose only child was at the point of death. The other was a woman, ceremonially unclean (an outcast of society), who had spent all of her money trying to be healed.

Jairus's Daughter

Jairus was a ruler of the synagogue whose chief function was conducting divine worship and arranging for those who would lead the various parts of the service. He did not allow his important position or his pride to stand in the way of admitting his need. Jairus was a desperate man looking for the one hope that would save his daughter. He turned to Jesus and asked him to come to his house and heal his twelve-year-old dying daughter. But before Jesus could proceed to the house, a woman with a hemorrhage touched him, and he stopped to heal her.

We can imagine Jairus's anxiety as he waited for Jesus, fearing that his daughter might die before he could arrive. While Jesus was still speaking to the woman, a servant came from Jairus's house to report that the daughter was dead. However, Jesus immediately reassured the father that if he had faith, his daughter would be healed.

When Jesus arrived at Jairus's house, the professional mourners were already wailing. This tradition may seem ostentatious and unnecessary to us, but in ancient Palestine hiring mourners showed respect for the dead. As he entered the house, Jesus told the mourners and friends not to weep anymore because the girl was asleep. He did not mean, humanly speaking, that she was alive; her death was not permanent because she would be awakened by Christ's miraculous power.

Because the raising of the dead girl was an intimate, tender moment, not a spectacular show, he allowed only his three closest disciples and her parents to come into the room. The precaution reflected his extreme thoughtfulness so that the girl would not wake up terrified in a room full of strangers. He took the child by the hand and tenderly told her to get up, and she arose immediately. The phrase used here by Luke—"her spirit returned"—is the same phrase used for Samson's revival of flagging power (Judg. 15:19); in other words, life returned to her.

We can imagine the astonishment of her parents. In fact they were so amazed, Jesus had to remind them to give her something to eat. He also did this to break the same sense of awe and terror that her death naturally would have created. Her mother certainly must have welcomed the opportunity to do something concrete and practical. Furthermore, it was proof that she was completely well and would follow a normal life.

Jesus' parting words to the parents were to tell no one about this miracle. First, he did not want the child to become the object of idle curiosity. Second, he did not want the event to lose its deep spiritual significance; they were to remain quietly with their daughter so that the miracle would not dissipate into gossip.

The Woman with the Hemorrhage

It is amazing that while Jesus was on the way to heal the daughter of a very important man in the community, he should take the time to heal a woman who was an outcast. The woman had had a hemorrhage for twelve years, which made her ritually unclean according to the Jewish laws of that time (Lev. 15). She could not be allowed to take part in any religious ceremonies, could not touch anyone, and would be separated from her husband. Furthermore, according to Mark's account, she had spent all her money on physicians in a vain attempt to be cured.

She had a partial and somewhat superstitious understanding of Jesus' power to heal; she believed it was necessary to touch part of his garment to be cured. The Hebrew concept of personality extended to the shadow, footprints, and clothes, so her belief was not especially unusual.

Because she wanted to be as inconspicuous as possible, she awaited an opportunity in the midst of the thronging crowd to touch his robe. (All devout Jews wore robes with fringes as a reminder that they were men of God committed to keeping the laws of God [Num. 15:37–41; Deut. 22:12].) She was healed immediately, and Jesus perceived that power had gone forth from him. She was frightened and nervous when Jesus asked who had touched him, but she came forward. She was given the opportunity to voluntarily come forward and confess publicly that Jesus had healed her. He did that in order for her healing to be complete. First, if her cure had taken place without its being publicly known, she would not have been accepted back into the community. Second, he wanted her to understand that it was not the touching of his garment that healed her, but her trust in him. When she confessed what had happened, the testimony in itself would strengthen her faith. Third, not only was her hemorrhage healed by the physical encounter, but her salvation was effected by the personal encounter of trust.

The Relationship between Faith and Healing

Both stories deal with the relationship between faith and healing. The faiths of both the woman and Jairus were imperfect. The woman supposed the power of Christ was really magical and mechanical. She was filled with superstitions, but Jesus used her faith to lead her to a higher understanding. He wanted her to know that faith depended on him and that only after a public confession could she receive the assurance of wholeness—both physical and spiritual.

The faith of Jairus was less superstitious than the woman's but fell short of the centurion's who did not even feel it was necessary for Jesus to come to his house to heal his servant. (See later discussion of the centurion.) However, Jairus's faith was tested and refined. First, he had to bear the news that his daughter was dead. His friends at that point told Jesus not to go to the house. Jairus, however, trusted Christ and followed him into his daughter's room.

Jesus asked for trust from those healed. But in neither of these healing miracles did he demand that first they be pure. He met them where they were and used the occasion for their spiritual growth.

The Paralyzed Man and His Friends

The story of the paralyzed man is recorded in Matthew 9:1–8, Mark 2:1–12, and Luke 5:17–26. Each account gives a unique emphasis. Luke was primarily interested in Jesus' healing power. The story took place while Jesus was teaching in a packed house where even the Pharisees and lawyers were present. A group of men were anxious for Jesus to heal their friend, but they had no way to get through the crowd, so they devised a very clever scheme of lowering him through the roof. Going through the roof was not as extraordinary as it might seem, since the Palestinian houses had flat roofs. They were composed of beams laid across with a twig and mortar mixture between them. Hence, the packing between the beams could be lifted out and the pallet lowered into the room.

Jesus did not register any surprise, but concentrated on the great faith of the friends. The man's illness was readily seen by everyone; the Greek word for paralysis indicates a disease of some part of the nervous system that meant he could do nothing but lie in bed. His body was disabled, but Jesus saw as well that his soul needed to be healed. First, Jesus forgave his sins, then the man could walk. The Levites and Pharisees, as usual, were upset with Jesus. They wondered what right he had to forgive sins. However, the man's ability to walk was proof that his sins were forgiven, so the Pharisees were speechless. The crowds were amazed at all the events, and news of Jesus' powers spread throughout the area.

The Role of Friends in Sickness

This miracle emphasizes that friends are very important when someone is sick. The friends had tremendous faith that they put into action. There was no need for them to be great talkers; they acted out their trust in Christ's power. Without their compassionate love, intercession, undaunted faith, and ingenious actions the man never would have been healed. Christ recognized at once their faith and healed the man. What a contrast to Job's friends, who were judgmental talkers; the paralyzed man's friends were sympathetic facilitators.

The Confusion of Sickness and Sin

The Pharisees were operating from a theology that equated sin and sickness, that is, if a person was suffering, he had sinned. They were incredulous at Jesus' audacity in claiming to forgive the man's sin since only God could do that. They were so blind about what was happening because they believed God should heal only through "regular" channels. They had not learned to look for the unexpected. Instead of recognizing Jesus as God, they accused him of blasphemy. Jesus clearly proved his right to forgive by also curing the man's paralysis. By their own argument the man was ill because he had sinned; his ability to walk was proof that his sins were forgiven.

The Paralyzed Man's Reaction

The story provides few details about the man; he was probably quite young because the word Jesus used in addressing him meant "child" or "my son," reflecting the love and pity Jesus felt for him. Although from the text, it is unclear if "their" faith refers to that of his friends or the man's, he did have a degree of trust.

He was willing to admit his need and to rely on his friends. One of the most difficult trials of being sick is the necessity of depending on other people. He allowed his friends to carry him to this self-proclaimed teacher for healing even to the point of being lowered through the roof. Talk about being the center of attention! He obeyed Jesus exactly; he did not argue that he had no sins to be forgiven. When he was commanded to get up off his bed, even though he was completely paralyzed, he not only got up; he also picked up his bed. He was extremely grateful for what Jesus had done, glorifying God to everyone he met.

Forgiveness and Healing

Jesus immediately perceived a connection between the man's sin and paralysis. His first act was to offer forgiveness so that healing could take place. No request had been made for such forgiveness, but Jesus saw into the heart of the man and saw his suffering of soul as well as body. In cases where sin causes sickness, the first and most important thing is forgiveness. Jesus did not give the man a lecture on his past life, but gave him the opportunity to start anew. The fact that Jesus could forgive sins was proof of his divinity and an expression of his love. He desired to deliver the man from the power of guilt and his bodily suffering.

No universal principle should be abstracted from this story that the forgiveness of sins must precede healing. However, examining our inner state, asking for forgiveness, may bring unexpected physical healing.

Real repentance is difficult because sin blocks us from God's power and hurts Christ. A great deal of time is often spent justifying our wrongdoing and calling on God only in extreme emergencies. Sometimes one harbors sins of which one is unaware and thinks that everything is all right. Real humility is needed for true repentance. When one is completely pardoned and can accept it, then guilt is removed. Often tension, hatred, resentment, bitterness, and unhappiness can bring severe physical pain. If these are removed through God's love, physical healing may take place. Forgiveness does not always bring freedom from physical illness, but inner healing does occur.

The Healing of the Centurion's Servant

The healing of the centurion's servant (Luke 7:1–10) took place at Capernaum, where Christ initiated his healing ministry. The centurion was a non-Jew, but was attracted to Judaism (Luke 7:5). He was probably a soldier in the service of Antipas. He sent a delegation asking Jesus to heal one of his beloved servants who was very ill. Jesus received the request and was on his way to the centurion's house. Just at that point another delegation arrived with the message that it was not necessary for Jesus to come but only to speak a word to heal the servant.

The centurion was obviously a man of great faith and deep humility. He did not think that he was worthy of a visit from the great rabbi and prophet. As a soldier he understood authority and realized that if a command was issued, obedience would follow. He believed that Jesus had authority over all people and unseen powers so that he could heal the servant simply by his spoken word. What was the basis of his great faith? No doubt he had heard about Jesus' miracles, particularly that of the healing of the nobleman's son (John 4), and he believed in his power.

Jesus praised the great faith of the centurion and responded to his request to heal his servant from a distance. The man was not only healed, but restored to complete health (as reflected by the Luke text).

The Son of the Widow of Nain

Jesus was always busy, and mobs of people usually followed him. After he healed the centurion's servant, the crowd no doubt grew even larger. Although the next miracle was recorded only in Luke, that does not undermine its authenticity. Numerous miracles were never recorded in detail (Luke 4:40–41; 6:18–19; John 2:23; 4:45). Those that were described most likely illustrated a specific point about Christ's healing message.

This miracle is a clear indication that Christ's healings were not a means to an end, or lesson materials for the crowds, but they welled up from Jesus' compassion for the people. As he was walking to Nain, to the southwest of Capernaum, a funeral procession was passing with a widow and her only son, who had died. She did not ask Jesus for anything, but he was touched by her sorrow and told her not to weep. He would naturally speak to her first because she was walking in front of the bier followed by hired mourners, musicians, and friends. He touched the bier so the procession would stop, then by his command brought the boy back to life. In all instances, Christ's command caused the raising of the dead (Luke 8:54; John 11:43). There is no mention of faith being involved in the healing either by the mother or by the boy, but simply the power of God. The crowd knew the miracle could only be the work of a prophet or God, and the news of the miracle spread all over Judea (Luke 7:11–17).

JESUS PROVIDES A PARADIGM FOR HEALING

These and other miracles form the focus of Jesus Christ's healing ministry, which provides a paradigm for healing. Four emphases in Jesus' healing ministry illumine the Christian perspective on the nature and process of healing: (1) Jesus affirms health as an important goal, desired by God; (2) he addresses the whole person while respecting his or her autonomy; (3) he meets people's voiced needs; and (4) he addresses what is behind a person's sickness. These emphases in Christ's healing ministry provide insight into the Christian ministry of healing.

Health Is a Central Goal

Contrary to some versions of later Christian piety, rather than acquiescing to sickness and suffering, Jesus overthrew them. His reactions in the face of sickness were pity and kindness (*splagchnizomai;* Mark 1:41; John 11:33), anger and indignation (*embrimaomai;* Matt. 9:30; Mark 14:5; John 11:33). Although he did not heal every sick person, the occasions on which he did heal make it clear that healing and health are central to God's work. It was—and is—not God's will for someone to suffer from illness. "Far from accepting sickness as the will of God, Jesus regarded his own healings as signs of God's power breaking in upon the kingdom of evil."[4] Not that one will experience in this life the full proportions of Christ's victory. Every person inevitably weakens, sickens, and dies. Jesus recognizes the limitations of human existence. However, Jesus' healing miracles are signs of life abundant and foreshadow the eternity promised through Christ's resurrection.

Jesus Addresses the Whole Person

Jesus sees and addresses us as autonomous in our situation. His healing acts are part of the transference of all of one's existence into a new dimension. His healing was not just a reconciliation of a person within himself or herself but with the whole of creation. Christ's preaching and healing ministry demonstrate the importance of physical health as well as spiritual wholeness. The human being does not vaporize into a disembodied spirit. Christ came not merely to save souls, but also to bring freedom and physical well-being. The health of body and spirit is part of God's perfect plan. The doctrine of the incarnation insists on the participation of the body in the work of salvation. God became human not only to suffer with humanity, but to be an example of what humanity was meant to be—whole persons, free and well.

Not everyone in the ancient world agreed with Jesus' concern for the whole person. Early Christians had to fight the Gnostic influences of their day, which regarded the body as evil, as reflected in their ascetic ethic. Gnostics repudiated the reality of Jesus' incarnation and bodily nature. The apostle Paul, who fought the Gnostic point of view, recognized the importance of a person's total being when he referred to the body as the temple of the Holy Spirit (1 Cor. 6:19). Paul's doctrine of the resurrection of the body reflected the understanding of salvation of the whole person. (See 1 Corinthians 15:35–38.)

Christ emphasized the whole person, yet he did not overwhelm the autonomy of the individuals he healed if they were interested in responding to him on only one level. Several stories illustrate this point. Jesus did not make the healing of the ten men with leprosy dependent upon their seeking a more complete healing. Only one of them evinced a desire for complete healing.

Similarly, Jesus showed respect for the patient when he asked the paralyzed man at the pool of Bethesda if he wanted to be healed (John 5:1–18). This healing occurred on the Sabbath during the Feast of Purim. (Observed in late winter, this feast celebrated the freeing of the Jews, by the action of Queen Esther, from Persian anti-Semitism. The day was marked by works of kindness and gift giving.) At the Sheep Gate at a pool with five porches called Bethesda (house of grace) or Beth-zatha (house of the olive), numerous sick people waited for the waters to move in order to be healed (John 5:7). Most likely, scores of sick people on blankets and pallets crowded around the pool, waiting eagerly in the hope of being healed. Among the crowd was the disabled man, ill for thirty-eight years—helpless and hopeless. He attracted Jesus' concern.

Jesus knew he had been sick for a long time and asked him, "Do you want to be made well?" (v. 6). (The word translated "made well" means both physical wellness and wholeness.) Behind Christ's question might have been the perception that, liking the attention his illness provided, the disabled man really did not want to be healed. Forthwith, Christ gave him a threefold command: "Stand up, take your mat and walk" (v. 8). The first command to stand tested his faith. Then he was commanded to carry his bed, his identifying mark, as proof of his complete recovery. He would be free of his past dependency as symbolized by the mat, and he would have no provision for falling back into his old way of living. The third command, "walk" (literally, "go on walking"), emphasized his entering into a new life and his continuing to live as a healed person. The force of "he walked" in the original Greek carries with it not only the idea of continual movement but perhaps the fulfillment that came from his recovered power. The man obeyed Jesus' command and was healed.

Even though Jesus must have realized the danger of being identified with the man, who by carrying his mat had broken the Sabbath law, Jesus sought him out in the Temple. As Jesus talked, the man began to understand healing in a larger light—not just of the body, but of the whole being. Apparently, Jesus was afraid that the man's bodily health might free him to sin further. It is unclear how his sickness was connected with his sin, but a connection was certainly implied. Jesus was not satisfied with giving him physical health but wanted to challenge him to strive against sin. His concern certainly supports the understanding that healing is much more than a restoration to physical health; spiritual well-being is even more important. When physical pain and disability are gone, our other problems still may remain.

Equally important in Jesus' approach was his requirement of responsible action by the sick person. Healing involved a decision by the paralyzed man to take hold of life. He was not allowed to indulge in simple resignation in the face of pain and illness.

A Healing Ministry Responds to Perceived Needs

Jesus met people where they were and moved them to where they should be. He also anticipated people's total needs if they were too debilitated by the effect of illness to verbalize them. The story of Bartimaeus, the blind beggar, illustrates this point (Mark 10:46–52).

Jesus was going to Jerusalem to celebrate the Passover. The crowds were large since it was a time of national pilgrimage to Jerusalem. One way to the city led through the Jordan Valley and then west through Jericho. Many were anxious to see Jesus, the audacious young Galilean who had stood up against the orthodox religious leaders of the day—forgiving sins, healing on the Sabbath, and preaching that the realm of God was at hand.

In the crowd gathered along that dusty road out of Jericho was a blind beggar, apparently well known in the area. When he heard all the noise and commotion, he asked what was happening. Upon learning that Jesus was passing by, he cried out, "Jesus, Son of David, have mercy on me!" (Mark 10:47). Bartimaeus's cry echoed the growing popular belief that Jesus was the messiah.

The crowd thought that Bartimaeus had no business bothering Jesus. They probably surmised he was asking for alms and should not trouble the famous rabbi. They rebuked him, but he was not put off and he called out even louder. By that time, Jesus heard him and called him forward. Reproofs were at once turned into encouragements as the crowd urged him to go forward.

His response to Jesus was immediate and eager. Mark added the vivid touches, omitted in the later Matthew and Luke accounts, that he cast away his cloak and sprang up (Mark 10:50). Throwing away his cloak was evidence of his complete trust in Jesus because a beggar's cloak was at once his bed, overcoat, and money receptacle.

Jesus asked him what he wanted. Bartimaeus knew exactly what he wanted—he wished to see and was not afraid to ask. Jesus not only opened his eyes but also commended him for his faith. The word *sozo,* translated "has made you whole" (Mark 10:52), includes the deeper sense of "saved," as mentioned earlier. Bartimaeus's theology might have been inadequate, for he perceived Jesus as a political king, but his instinctive response and trust in Christ were much more important. His firm expectancy was a channel through which the healing grace of Jesus Christ could pass. Moreover, he did not selfishly go off on his own once his need was met. Having received his sight, he followed Jesus "on the way" (a technical term in the Christian Scriptures for becoming a disciple).

This story illustrates how Christ's ministry responded to needs as they were presented, but also moved a person past those needs to a broader vision of a changed life. Jesus met people at the point of their particular need. In some cases, it was a physical ailment—leprosy, blindness, deafness, or paralysis. In other cases, the disorder was moral, for example, the rich young ruler who did not want to give up his possessions. What marked Jesus' healing was his attitude of caring; the relationship between Jesus and the person he was healing was of paramount importance. One of the terms used to describe Jesus as a healing agent is *diakonia,* translated either "ministry" or "service." Wholeness was effected in various ways: teaching, preaching, healing, washing feet, forgiving, comforting, and so forth.[5]

Jesus Addresses What Underlies a Person's Sickness

The story of the healing of the paralyzed man (Matt. 9:1–8; Mark 2:1–12; Luke 5:17–26), discussed earlier, illustrates Christ's concern not only to cure, but also to address the problems underlying illness. Jesus was interested in changing people's health-defeating patterns. His healings were gifts offered without requirements. However, by giving some instructions to those being healed, he moved them beyond sickness to its cause. He called people to repentance, to move away from the things that brought disintegration and division into their lives. He regarded them not as passive victims, but as active agents responsible for their own health. Jesus' call was to restoration of function or restoration of equilibrium, and also conviction to a life of love and service. Sacrificing one's life for others completes what it means to be whole ("For those who want to save their life will lose it, and those who lose their life for my sake, and for the sake of the gospel, will save it" [Mark 8:35]).

In light of Christ's healing ministry, is it possible to refer to Jesus as a physician? Given the contemporary use of the term, that would be misleading. However, if a broader definition is employed, "a person skilled in the art of healing," then Jesus exemplifies what a physician should be.[6] Christ is the healer par excellence. Christ teaches about healing and about how to be healers. He used no set formula or method. Furthermore, no diseases are beyond the power of God when we trust in God's power. Nevertheless, not everyone was healed by Jesus. We are left with the mystery of suffering in the face of the love of God, while still affirming the importance of physical health from Christ's perspective. As one delves deeply into Christ's healing ministry, it provides a foundation for starting one's own healing ministries.

MIRACULOUS HEALING

At the center of the discussion of Christ's healing ministry is the question of miraculous healing. Why does God not eliminate suffering by a miracle? Do miracles still happen? What is meant by the term? Should one pray for and claim miracles? Do miracles result only from faith, or do they come by means of medicine and drugs?

Many people view miracles as arbitrary interventions of God into the world. However, as Augustine pointed out centuries ago, miracles are not occurrences contrary to nature; they are contrary only to the known processes of nature. God does not arbitrarily change the course of nature, but events that appear to be miracles actually demonstrate the complexity and majesty of the natural world and increase our understanding and awe of God's power. Further, miracles give clues to the nature of God's work in the total process of salvation—cleansing, liberating, and restoring. Miracles, therefore, function as signs. A helpful definition of miracles is that they are God's divine surprises.

In writing about the ante-Nicene fathers' view of the healing ministry, Evelyn Frost rightly points out the danger of discarding all elements of the Christian faith that do not match rational approaches to knowledge. Frost argues for miraculous healing to be put in a sphere of the "unrationalized as yet" and left there pending further knowledge. God's workings may not be ultimately understandable; human explanations are mere guesses as to how God's laws function.[7] As Denis Duncan points out, Christopher Cooke argued against the use of the word "intervention" and for God's "continuing creation" when referring to a miracle. This emphasizes the ongoing creative activity of God; these events belong to knowledge that is "beyond knowledge."[8] I personally experienced the inexplicable when my two-year-old son fell straight down a three-story stairwell in our apartment in Basel, Switzerland, and suffered only a large lump on his head. The physician summoned to examine him stated, *"Das ist nicht ein medizinisches problem, aber ein theologisches problem."* ("This is not a medical problem, but a theological problem.")

Many writers prefer to limit the term "miracle" solely to Christ's activity. Others eliminate the word "miracle" altogether after the apostolic age and refer instead to these unexplainable events as signs of "God's mighty works." They react against defining miracles as events that reveal laws of nature not yet understood. The concern is that later when an explanation for a miracle is found, it shakes the definition of miracle.[9] The difficulty here is tracing cause and effect. Should one name "spontaneous cures" or "remissions" as miracles?

Form criticism of the Scriptures has become the basis for many scholars to expunge accounts of miracles from the Bible. Maddocks, in discussing the form critics' approach to Jesus' healing miracles, suggests one should place the miracles in three categories: the Isaianic signs, the exorcisms, and the theological parable-miracles. Form criticism eliminates some miracles, but still miraculous healings are attested by Scripture.[10]

In the Hebrew and Christian Scriptures, miracles are grouped around particular periods of history. Miracles are recorded during the events leading up to the exodus from Egypt in the book of Exodus and during the lifetimes of Elijah and Elisha. The biblical writers were concerned not with whether events as miracles were contrary to nature but how they reflected God's control and power in the world. Miracles were accepted as such by the faithful. Even if a miracle is eventually explained, the sense of God's power and presence does not disappear for the believer.[11]

To understand the biblical writers' accounts, we need to examine the theology behind them. For the Hebrews, nature does not govern itself apart from God. God is expressed through nature, and not in opposition to it. Furthermore, later finding an explanation for an extraordinary event does not necessarily eliminate its function as a sign. Ultimately, faith alone assesses an event as miraculous. A miracle points to its source, God. God's grace and power energize the whole system of nature, which brings healing. Health is viewed as mainly in God's hands.

The most explicit accounts of healing through an agent of God are in the Elijah-Elisha cycles of 1 and 2 Kings: the story of Elijah's healing of the widow's son (1 Kings 17), Elisha's restoration to life of the son of the Shunammite woman (2 Kings 4), and Elisha's cure of Naaman's leprosy (2 Kings 5). These are all understood as evidence of God's control over history.[12]

God is described as the healer (Exod. 15:25–26). The early Exodus chapters recount how God punishes the evildoers but rewards those who follow God's commandments. So the Egyptians are sent diseases and plagues, and the Israelites are saved from such punishment. The image of healing is often used in relation to God and Israel. "I kill and I make alive; I wound and I heal; and no one can deliver from my hand" (Deut. 32:39). Throughout the book of Hosea, the question is raised, Who will heal Israel? The image that Ezekiel uses in his prophecy of renewal is one of healing.

The use of the term "signs and wonders" in the Hebrew Scriptures did not indicate healings; rather, it referred to God's deliverance of the Israelites from various perils. Even in Isaiah 35 with the description of eschatological healings ("the eyes of the blind shall be opened, and the ears of the deaf unstopped; then the lame shall leap"), the events were not understood as "signs and wonders," which is the definition of miracles in the Christian Scriptures. It is interesting that Jesus quoted this passage to John's disciples when they wondered if he was the Messiah (Luke 7:22).

In the Christian Scriptures, miracles are grouped in two main periods, that is, during Christ's ministry and after Pentecost. The purpose of the miracles was to confirm that Christ was indeed the Messiah and that the apostles were true heirs of Jesus as they displayed the same powers that he had.

A miracle is a symbol as well as an event in the Christian Scriptures. Miracles revealed something about the nature of Jesus. They symbolize the divine mercy that broods over human life and the divine dimension to life that is the source of renewing power. Jesus' miracles were signs of new life. God's power broke into time and space. Faith reveals an open universe, an open system that scientists as well as theologians may grasp. During the controversies of nineteenth-century rationalism, the miracles in the Christian Scriptures were rejected as not fitting into a closed view of the universe. As science has advanced, however, especially one's understanding of psychology and psychosomatic medicine, and a post-Newtonian physics, miracles seem more believable.

In the Christian Scriptures, Christ's miracles reveal God's work. The three words for miracle in the Christian Scriptures reflect its different dimensions: "wonders," "signs," and "powers." The wonders (*teras;* Acts 2:22) indicated the state of mind that a miracle produced in eyewitnesses. They drew attention to God and God's purposes.

Signs (*sēmeion*) had as their most prominent element their ethical purpose; they were a pledge of what was to come. They allowed one set of facts to signify the reality, genuineness, and nature of the more ultimate set of events of which they were a part. They revealed Jesus Christ's true glory and corroborated his claim to be the Child of God and deepened the faith of those who heard him speak (Matt. 8:27; 9:7; Mark 7:37; Luke 13:17; John 2:11; 14:11; 20:30–31). In answering the question of John's disciples if he was the messiah, Jesus referred to his physical healings:

> When the men had come to him, they said, "John the Baptist has sent us to you to ask, 'Are you the one who is to come, or are we to wait for another?'" Jesus had just then cured many people of diseases, plagues, and evil spirits, and had given sight to many who were blind. And he answered them, "Go and tell John what you have seen and heard: the blind receive their sight, the lame walk, the lepers are cleansed, the deaf hear, the dead are raised, the poor have good news brought to them." (Luke 7:20–22)

The third word, *dunamis* (powers), from which our word "dynamite" comes, refers to the cause of miracles, that is, the power of God. These are events wrought by the direct power of God. God is the source of all healing and it is the Creator's power that restores us to wholeness. This power, at a certain moment in history, was directed through one man; all healing put on a face and hands in the person of Jesus.

Apart from these references, the Christian Scriptures have little else to say about healing except in the Pauline passage in 1 Corinthians 12 and in James 5:13–20. The latter passage seems more concerned about prayer than healing per se and refers to a certain type of prayer service for healing.[13]

As one moves from the time of the Christian Scriptures, the view of miraculous healing becomes even more unclear. There are two schools of thought about the place of miraculous healing in the life of the church. The more traditional Protestant view is that they ceased with the apostolic age, according to studies by William Warfield in *Miracles: Yesterday and Today, True and False.*[14] In the patristic writings, first-century "exorcisms" were prevalent but not miraculous healings. They next appear in the later days of Augustine (400 C.E.), when miracle-working shrines were cited. (Here one might wonder if this was in fact due to the peasants' superstitious belief in shrines and wooded places that were purported to hold special power rather than stemming from Christian theology.) What is clear is that God is not limited in the way God heals; miracles do happen.

Apostolic Healing

Christ's healing ministry also illustrates that individual Christians are called to be healing agents in other people's lives. The church is the corporate expression of the individual Christian's calling to a healing ministry. Christ sent disciples to preach, teach, and heal: "He called the twelve and began to send them out two by two, and gave them authority over the unclean spirits. . . . So they went out and proclaimed that all should repent. They cast out many demons, and anointed with oil many who were sick and cured them" (Mark 6:7, 12–13). Since Christ's mission included the care of persons' bodies as well as their spirits, it is not surprising that healing was such a critical part of the mission of the Twelve. No other prophet, not even Moses or Elijah, gave miraculous powers to his disciples.

The apostles were given this ministry of healing for three reasons: (1) Jesus Christ healed; (2) they were to share his compassion; and (3) they were to act in accordance with the gospel they were preaching. Christ spent a major portion of his time in healing. Jesus' motive for healing was his compassion. Hence, the disciples were not to be impelled by monetary gain or to make a trade of their miraculous powers. Their cures were not ends in themselves, but were to lend support to and to clarify the meaning of the gospel message of God's saving love.

Jesus gave his apostles the power and authority to perform miracles. First, they would cast out demons. (The obedience of the demons was a sign of the disciples' conquest of Satan, the prince of demons [Luke 10:17–18].) In addition, they were to cleanse people who had leprosy, heal people who were sick, and raise people who were dead. Christ did not give them one particular methodology for healing, though the use of oil is specifically mentioned (Mark 6:13). The medicinal use of oil was common in the ancient world (see Isa. 1:6; Luke 10:34), but among the disciples it was most likely a symbolic practice. It appears later in the church (James 5:14) and finally in the Roman Catholic Church as a sacramental rite.

The healing ministry was passed from the disciples to the apostles. Acts contains the story of the further missionary work (preaching and healing) of the apostles, especially Peter and Paul. The apostle Paul listed healing among the gifts of the Holy Spirit (1 Cor. 12:30). Peter's healing of the disabled man showed that the disciples took seriously Christ's command to heal. That was followed by the preaching of the Word as the two acts went together (Acts 4). Other stories illustrate their healing ministry: Aeneas, who was cured (Acts 9:34); Tabitha, who was raised from the dead (Acts 9:36–43); and Paul's healing of the man who was unable to walk (Acts 14:8–10). Healings are also described on the island of Malta (Acts 28:1–10).[15] Additional passages describe the healing of the multitudes. These healings reflect the power of the Holy Spirit that filled Christ's apostles, giving credence and authority to their message. The epistle of James indicates that the leaders of the church regularly exercised a ministry to the sick by the laying on of hands and the anointing with oil (James 5:13–18).

Faith healing and even miraculous healing have reemerged not only in the church but in society in general. In fact, these topics have been featured in several popular magazines describing how disenchantment with scientific medicine, as well as a recognition of the inexplicable remissions of illness, has created a new openness to the importance of faith. In some ways, the traditional churches may lag behind society in embracing faith healing. This probably is related to concerns about the dangers described at the beginning of this chapter. Reviewing Christ's healing ministry may have provided some insight on this subject as we move to the next part of the book, which focuses on healers and how we can all be agents of healing.

Part 3

Healers as Coadventurers for Health

8

The Patient
as the Central Healer

As we move from a consideration of the nature of healing, of prime importance are the roles and relationships of the professional healers to one another and to the patient. These are especially significant in light of what healers can do to relieve suffering and be instruments of healing.

If health is personal wholeness and healing refers to any activity that moves us toward wholeness, then anyone who contributes to our journey toward health is a healer. No one professional is responsible for all our health-related needs. The job of healing is bigger than any single profession or individual.

But if no one professional handles the whole person, how does one avoid dividing up the individual, hence losing the very integration that one is trying to achieve? The only solution seems to be to have the patient as the integrator. The patient is the central healer because other healers enter at the patient's initiative or in response to the patient's need. When the patient can no longer function completely as the central healer, she or he draws others into the circle.

Two Popular Models

There are two popular ways to see the patient as healer—first, through the physical fitness movements and, second, through the rise of self-help groups. One could describe the fitness culture as emerging from the 1960s counterculture vegetarians and natural food purists; this movement later was coupled with the medical community's concerns over cholesterol and sugar levels, and that was conjoined with the jogging and health spa phenomena. In short, flab and indulgence were supposedly replaced by the take-charge-of-my-body individual. According to some studies, however, these fitness phenomena touch very few Americans, and people actually weigh more than they did ten years ago.[1] Yet these approaches have little to do with an integrated approach to self-care. Furthermore, they are not unique to the current scene. For example, diet and exercise were part of Wesley's Methodism,[2] and in the late 1800s, practitioners of Social Catholicism such as Nichols emphasized them.[3] These concerns are somewhat similar to those of homeopathic and medical botanists of that period who were resistant to orthodox medicine.[4] Perspectives on the patient as healer are much broader.

Since the late 1950s, the self-help movement has been part of U.S. health care. In the 1960s and 1970s, according to John Stoeckle, the dominance of the medical profession created a focus on the body, not the person.[5] Hence, patients turned to one another for a more wholistic approach. Beginning with the founding of Alcoholics Anonymous in 1935, there has been a steady increase in the types of self-help groups in the United States and more and more research about their effectiveness. Much of this growth occurred after World War II, stimulated by the community mental health movement in the 1950s, the initiation of government programs in the 1960s, and the women's movement in the 1970s.

In the late 1980s and 1990s, there has been a tremendous resurgence of self-help, self-care groups. There are more than 820 types of self-help groups. A recent national survey estimated that between eight and ten million Americans belong to a self-help group and that there are approximately 500,000 individual groups in the country. The Midlife Development in the United States (MIDUS) estimate that twenty-five million Americans have participated in self-help groups at some time in their lives is likely to be con- servative because (1) the survey excluded people younger than twenty-five and older than seventy-five; and (2) the MIDUS's definition of a self-help group excludes groups either organized or led by professionals. Clearinghouse data suggest that a substantial proportion of support groups are, in fact, facil- itated by a professional. On the other hand, an estimated ten million Americans participated in a self-help group in 1996.[6] The increase of home testing and treatment technologies has strengthened the self-help movement. A growing body of research is emerging about self-help groups.

Self-help groups, aside from church school and Bible study groups, are the most prevalent formal support groups in the United States today. Self- help is now a major institution in U.S. society. Most self-help groups are small and local. The participants are more likely to be young, female, white, and unmarried. Clearly, if self-help is to be an effective accommodation to budget cuts in the human services system, the development of new models will be necessary.

A new interest in self-help groups has developed between clinicians and social policy analysts as financial constraints increasingly have restricted the range of services available to clients of the human services system. The largest single sector in the U.S. mental and addictive disorders treatment system is the self-help sector. There are self-help groups for people who have survived traumatic life experiences as well as for people grappling with various current life problems. More than one-third of participants—accounting for more than 70 percent of self-help meeting attendance—are involved in groups for substance use problems.

As important as self-help groups are, understanding how the patient assists in his own healing is much more comprehensive. The patient as healer deserves prime attention since other healers enter at his initiative or in response to his need. There are a number of advantages to the patient being the central healer: (1) he will take an active role in his own care, which itself brings healing; (2) he can decide who is most appropriately involved from the perspective of his value system and health needs, for example, a Christian Scientist would not want an internist or an atheist a pastor; (3) he can prevent paternalism by deciding the extent and type of professional involvement; and (4) he can more naturally involve nonprofessionals such as family, friends, and associates in his health care. The only problem with this approach is that if a person is debilitated by illness, where will he receive the strength and staying power to effect that integration? The patient seeks professionals precisely because he is in a state of need.

PATIENT'S DISCONTENT WITH PASSIVE ROLE

The general discontent with the medical model and the acceptance of the sick role may have as much to do with the passive role of the patient in her own healing as they do with any shortcomings of the medical profession. The patient defects from, or has taken away by the doctor, her responsibility and then reclaims this responsibility in an adversarial manner when things go wrong. If, however, she were substantively involved as one of the healers, she would bear at least partially the responsibility for the outcome. (Whether this would be relevant to the court proceedings is not known.) This is different from Illich's point that the medical profession robs the patient of power; the concern here is not with power but with responsibility.

It is difficult to recognize the patient as one of the healers since the word itself means "one who suffers or bears up." Cassell states, "It is a fundamental error to consider a sick person the same as a well person but with a disease stuck on the side—much as the person would carry a knapsack."[7] The ways of thinking, feeling, and living are altered, so no one should pretend that there are no changes. The debilitating effects of illness are manifold and impair the ability of patients to have perspective.[8] All events are interpreted as related to them: nurses are slow because they do not like them; doctors are short-tempered because they have done something wrong. Illness causes a patient's world to shrink, by reducing the resources available for his struggle to get well. The shattering psychological effects of the acknowledgment of disease often lead to its denial, though intuitively patients may sense when their illness is terminal. Patients become disconnected from their world and lose a sense of omnipotence. Their reactions to disease are primarily emotional and cause them to overlook obvious diagnoses.[9]

THE POWER INEQUALITY BETWEEN PATIENT AND PHYSICIAN

There are two possible responses by a physician to the patient's weakened state: (1) to take control of decision making for the patient; and (2) to abdicate any responsibility, pretending that the patient is the same as a well person. Neither option is appropriate. The doctor should "help the patient maintain his or her autonomy to the degree possible in the face of illness."[10]

Knowledge alone cannot bridge the basic inequality between the physician and the patient. This inequality stems primarily from the patient's dependency that, for Cassell, is a necessary state of illness. This dependency creates a willingness to receive what is important for the patient-physician relationship. While the patient is needy, the physician appears omnipotent. Pellegrino, citing Selzer, also describes the inequality of power in this relationship.[11]

It is questionable whether Cassell's analysis is completely accurate, for physical illness need not alter one's self-image. For example, as Kass has suggested, the physicist who has to use a wheelchair may be more whole than the stress-driven, chain-smoking corporate president. Leon Eisenberg has shrewdly observed that patienthood might be more a psychological than a biological state. In fact, community studies indicate that some 75 to 90 percent of episodes self-identified as illness are managed entirely without recourse to a medical system.[12]

The designation of the patient as healer follows from the definition of health as wholeness and the recognition of healing as any activity that moves one on the road to wholeness. A twofold theological basis exists for the patient as healer: (1) the dignity and worth of each person as a locus of value that illness cannot alter; and (2) the responsibility of each person to be a steward of creation, including oneself.

The centrality of the patient as healer is not arbitrarily asserted, but theologically grounded in the dignity and equality of all persons. This worth depends not upon the degree of knowledge or expertise of the individual, but upon her inherent value as a child of God. Furthermore, the patient should be viewed as a moral agent with ethical responsibilities. Truth telling and confidentiality are not injunctions only to the doctor.

Although one must readily acknowledge that illness may create a partial impotence to exercise the functions of humanhood, it does not necessarily create an impotence to be a person. An individual's value is not contingent upon health. Furthermore, one should relate to people in terms of health and wholeness, not sickness and brokenness. (This parallels the treatment of persons with disabilities when the focus is incorrectly on their disabilities rather than on them as individuals.) "Hence it seems to be a fundamental demand of the ethics of the sickbed that the sick person should not cease to let himself be addressed and to address himself, in terms of health, and the will which it requires rather than sickness, and above all to see to it that he is in an environment of health."[13]

Viewing the patient, not first as broken or diseased, but as a precious individual, mandates contesting disease and fighting sickness as the intrusion of death into the stream of life.[14] Furthermore, this view recognizes that a person is not just a body, but has a spiritual side to his or her nature.

THE CHARGE TO BE ONE'S OWN HEALER

The responsibility for one's own health—the charge to be, in part, one's own healer—stems from one's calling as a steward of creation; that is, to be a caretaker, overseeing the proper use of the gifts of creation including one's body.[15] One of the most important contributions of the Christian church to a health and healing ministry is the education of individuals to treat their bodies as the temple of the Holy Spirit, hence caring for themselves by pursuing healthy lifestyles. What one does for and to oneself can be twice as powerful as all the benefits of technomedicine. There is fertile ground for the church community to take a leadership role in developing a commitment to community health. The church can become a healing community by providing individuals with the knowledge and motivation to enhance their health and that of the community.[16] The body has its own healing power, for example, the scarring of the body in response to a wound. One of the least recognized and important truths about health care is that it cannot actually be delivered. The key to health is personal responsibility. People exercise this responsibility when they adopt patterns and habits of life that promote good health.

The active role of the patient is an essential factor in explaining why healing occurs in some cases and not in others. As the patient teaches, he also becomes a healer. These two roles of teacher and healer merge when patients participate in decisions about their treatment. A widely known example is that of Norman Cousins, who devised his own rather unorthodox treatment, after consultation with his physician, of laughter and vitamin C for a serious collagen illness, which is a disease of the connective tissue.[17]

Medical technologies provide the removal of the obstacles to becoming healthy, for example, cleaning a wound and applying antibiotics. The physician brings skills to minimize impairment of physical functions. However, the first rule of medicine is *primum non nocere*, emphasizing the body's powers for regeneration and the importance of the physician's doing nothing to impede the natural healing process. This fact may explain the faith healer's "success" since the faith of the patient may enable the body's natural regenerative powers to work.

One respects one's life and dignity as one adopts a life discipline that enhances health and well-being. Following patterns that have been identified as healthy—balanced diet, exercise, no smoking, alcohol in moderation, use of seat belts, and adequate sleep—reflects a sense of self-worth as well as care of one's whole being.

Motivation to Be a Healer

Any discussion of the patient as healer must pose the issue of motivation to assume that role. There are three aspects to this motivation: (1) to work to keep well, (2) to want to get well if sick, and (3) to take an active role in becoming well. The sick role brings privileges, such as freedom from personal and professional demands. For the mother of a large family or the business executive, the only release from the relentlessness of the routine may be illness. The attention received by family and friends may also be difficult to relinquish. If one has been starved for attention, one's illness may be the best vehicle for obtaining it. The story of Jesus' healing of the paralyzed man by the Bethesda pool acknowledges the hesitancy that some feel about the cost of becoming well.

However, people generally want to get well. Motivation to be well may stem from negative forces; sickness creates a tension that people naturally wish to avoid. When pain becomes great, it moves people to change and motivates them to growth and wholeness. The source of the pain may be emotional, physical, social, spiritual, or intellectual.[18] Positive motivation is more effective because it stems from a vision of what it means to be well and a desire to return to the task of living a full life.

Taking an active role in one's healing is often inhibited by a confusion between the nonvoluntary/nonculpable dimension of illness and the degree of patient responsibility. According to Parsons, U.S. culture emphasizes rest and relaxation—a passive relation to illness—rather than an active role in recovery, such as might have been observed in the older Russian culture.[19] People want to pay someone to make them well rather than work at preventing their illness.

The sick role can be rejected or embraced. For example, Siegler and Osmond describe the case of a middle-aged doctor who had an acute coronary heart attack and would not acknowledge his condition and stop working; hence he died twenty hours later. On the other hand, a seventeen-year-old with a brain tumor thought if he were "good" and followed all the doctor's instructions, he would be healed; he also died. Acknowledging the sick role may be important for entering treatment, but it may also raise false expectations regarding recovery or encourage a degree of passivity.

Understanding the patient's responsibility is a good counterpoint to passivity. There is a real reticence to make patients responsible for their own illness. It is believed to be judgmental and unfair. Yet by the same token, one is responsible for succeeding in one's professional career, producing creative works, and winning an athletic contest. On the other side, becoming obese, flunking an exam, or ruining a promising career may be laid at the feet of the individual. One does not shirk from referring to responsibility in these situations. Why should the same not be true for health and sickness? The point here is not some self-care movement where medical wisdom is set aside, but a collaborative style; taking responsibility enhances one's self-image and respect.

Confronting Self-Destructive Behaviors

Taking responsibility for one's own health is hard. Taking a pill or continuing in the same patterns is preferable to taking charge of our body, mind, and heart. Dealing with stress is a crucial part of taking responsibility for our health. It forces us to recognize our limitations to respond to everything, everybody, every expectation, and every need in the environment.

Identifying self-destructive behavior is also integral to moving toward health. Menninger in *Man against Himself* even goes so far as to say that illness is "a flight from frustration and the responsibilities of life."[20] Guilt-producing behavior and negative emotions throw the body into a precarious position, so natural barriers are down. Some believe that if the sick person is a patient, she can blame everyone else for what is happening to her. David Belgum pleads that we move from patient to penitent so that we can own our responsibility, hence recover.[21]

Patients who do not want to get well strongly inhibit the doctor's ability to heal them. Emotional states may lead to a wide variety of physical symptoms. Emotions of anger and frustration may lead to stomach ulcers, fear and anxiety may be forerunners of heart disease, persistent irritation may cause dermatitis, and unresolved grief may result in ulcerative colitis.[22] There are other studies on psychosomatic illnesses tracing the onset of cancer to grief, the pathogenic factor in rheumatoid arthritis, the emotional factors of sexual anxiety and jealousy in asthmatic attacks.[23]

One doctor has even said there are no incurable diseases, only incurable people. One must confront the destructive reality with resources of the spirit. Santayana said, "Nothing is inherently and invincibly young except spirit. And spirit can enter a human being perhaps better in the quiet of old age and dwell there more undisturbed than in the turmoil of adventure."[24]

The human spirit may help a patient develop the will to be well—an important step toward healing. If someone is starved for attention, illness may be the best vehicle for obtaining it. There may be some sickness that is the person's fault. Medically speaking, if a person has a wound, he has to admit he has a wound, then the doctor has to open it up and remove all foreign particles so that it can heal. This same principle is at work in mental and spiritual healing, which may need to precede physical healing.

Effects of Attitude and Activity

A patient can work at staying well by being positive. Unhappiness, doctors tell us, precedes many illnesses. Norman Cousins, as previously mentioned, proved the therapeutic value of laughter. John Pitch has stated that the key elements of wellness are knowing the purpose of life, understanding its genuine joys and pleasures, and assuming total and complete self-responsibility. A sense of humor can help even against the worst diseases. A very interesting study of college sophomores in the 1940s revealed a correlation between mental health and physical wellness. Investigators made periodic checks on physical and mental health. Poor mental health was a key predictor of early physical deterioration. Of the forty-eight men who had the worst mental health between ages twenty-one and forty-six, eighteen were hit with chronic illness or death by age fifty-three. That was independent of whether they smoked, drank, were overweight, or had parents who died young. George Valliant of the psychiatry department at Cambridge Hospital, Massachusetts, concludes, "No matter what, the men who were better at loving, who had more satisfying personal relations, seem to avoid early aging, while the health of poor emotional copers was significantly more likely to deteriorate during middle age."[25]

It is evident that an individual patient's ability to be a healer is determined to a large degree by the kind of person she is. A person who has faced other crises courageously may react optimistically to cancer compared with someone who has failed repeatedly in other challenges. Earlier success, however, does not guarantee victory. When illness no longer permits one to perform the past roles of mother or corporate president, a special kind of suffering results from the loss of personal identity. This suffering may produce a sense of hopelessness. It is precisely at this point that vibrant faith in God may sustain hope, whether it be of immediate cure or ultimate victory in eternity.

Furthermore, with the professionalization of society, one yields responsibility to the experts—believing the specialization and technical nature of knowledge preclude lay involvement in health care. Yet the active role of a patient's self-care and prevention may do more than anything else to change the face of contemporary medicine. This lay approach to self-care has always been at the heart of the nursing profession. For paraplegic, cerebral palsy, diabetic, and even kidney dialysis patients, self-care is not only possible but desirable. Self-care also forms one of the central tenets of the holistic health movement. According to Effie Poy Yew Chow (nurse, acupuncture practitioner, and former president of the East-West Academy of Healing Arts), holistic medicine emphasizes disease prevention and the individual as self-healer.[26] Self-care from this perspective does not refer to compliance with a physician's treatment program, but emphasizes the patient's resources for healing. For someone such as Elliott Dacher, who was chief of Georgetown University Community Health Plan in Reston, Virginia, self-care translates into wellness groups for patient support and education: "The greatest healer is inside and I don't think our doctors know our bodies better than we know them ourselves."[27]

Self-Care and Following Directions
Generally, we rely on physicians and drugs to rescue us from the effects of unhealthy lifestyles rather than take hold of ourselves and change destructive habits. Instead, the doctor should encourage, equip, and educate the patient as one of the healers, which, in Pellegrino's terms, is part of enhancing the moral agency of the patient. However, taking an active role in becoming well requires, at a minimum, compliance with recommended treatment. The patient who works with the physician to return to health heals faster than the uninterested or negative patient.

Understanding the patient as healer is not simply related to self-care or promotion of healthy lifestyles; it is also related to compliance with medical directives. This is a complex area to address because some medical prescriptions are ineffectual at best and illness-producing at worst. Even by seeking the advice of two or three specialists, one cannot always be sure of the facts of one's case or the best way to proceed. Having said all that, however, generally speaking if an individual chooses a trusted physician, it behooves the individual to follow the physician's recommendations for a return to health.

What influences a given patient to comply with a course of treatment is difficult to substantiate; studies available on this subject provide conflicting data. Variables related to treatment compliance have been grouped by illness and demographic, social, and psychological factors. For example, patients being treated for recurrent ulcers, who did not understand the reason for their treatment, expressed a fear of dying, and those who were critical toward physicians who had previously treated them were less likely to comply with requests.[28] In general, highly work-oriented patients are less compliant than less work-oriented patients. Catholics are more compliant than Protestants based on their respect for authority. Patients with average levels of anxiety remembered the doctor's instructions better than those with high or low anxiety.[29]

Important to healing is the patient's proactive role in recovery. The individual has partial responsibility for activating the body's mechanisms that not only protect from disease but engage the relevant antibodies when protections are breached. The patient's role is to pursue a healthy lifestyle and to share in choices and application of therapy.

The Effect of Faith

Choices in treatment will be influenced by one's value system, and recovery may be linked to one's personal faith. Studies at Johns Hopkins Medical Center illustrate that the faith factor is significant in a patient's recovery from a wide variety of illnesses.[30] It appears that the faith itself rather than the object of the faith is of primary importance.

The first element of faith is expectancy—the use of placebos with patients has shown that expectancy of improvement may actually produce improvement. Suggestion is another powerful force. If one expects to improve, one will. Personality type is also a factor. Usually, the religious person has a mood of expectancy, is more open to suggestion, is hopeful, and is able to relate to others in a life-modifying relationship.[31]

Cultivating a sense of hope about oneself and the course of one's illness is central to recovery. Hopelessness creates a sense of futility. If a particular goal is unachievable, then everything seems impossible, and frustration extends to every aspect of life. This response is natural in the face of serious and debilitating illness. If one's self-image is involved with prowess in sports, for example, then losing the ability to move one's legs may make all of life seem hopeless. Physical therapy and rehabilitation are avoided, and any improvement of health and strength is undermined. Regaining hope is central in a patient's becoming a healer—it involves a balance between emotional support to prevent self-destruction and the encouragement of the person to accept responsibility for his situation. Hope becomes grounded in a realistic appraisal of life.

Several new approaches from a Christian faith perspective involve patients in their healing and health care. One approach used at the Bethel Baptist healing ministry in Kingston, Jamaica, is a wholistic life chart for use by patients in their prayer life. It lists all the resources available to a person for healing of body, mind, and spirit, for example, material resources such as food, housing, work situation, neighbors, support groups, friends, and the church.[32]

Another ministry is that of a hospice—a hospital for the dying that creates a home environment founded by Cecily Saunders in London, England, and now finally established as part of the U.S. health care system. The emphasis is on the patient staying in control in the face of death and pain. A home is simulated with patients surrounded by loved ones. Freedom from control of pain that drains energies is also achieved, which enhances the quality of life. In fact, sometimes patients who go to a hospice to die recover and go home even if only for a few months.

Healing is more than medical factors. People are cured with or without medical professionals. Patients are important, but more studies are needed to determine their role as healers. How do patients interact with the physiological, psychological, spiritual, environmental, or community contributions to health and sickness?

The style of the traditional family doctor was wholistic in the limited sense of dealing with all aspects of the person in the family setting. The ideal of the family doctor, however, failed to regard the patient herself as a healer—responsible for her own health. Coupled with this perspective is the patient's teaching responsibility to the doctor. Pellegrino and Cassell discuss this responsibility in relation to selecting and evaluating proper treatment for a patient. The doctor does not bestow well-being/well-working; it is achieved as a result of one's active responsibility.

THE PATIENT AS TEACHER

Eric Cassell clearly delineated that the course of an illness is influenced by its host, so diagnosis and treatment are tied to knowledge of and from the patient. The patient is a teacher. He assists other healers by giving clear and accurate information. The subjective data from the patient about his illness are as important as the scientific information about the patient's disease.[33] Michael Balint in his landmark book *The Doctor, the Patient, and Illness* analyzed various cases with respect to the importance of the patient's assistance in arriving at an accurate diagnosis.[34] His work was the basic text for British medical students for decades. As Balint expressed it, the physician should "release the doctor that is within the patient." This does not reduce to the patient's recital of symptoms and an accurate case history, but sharing perceptions about the course of one's disease and one's responsibility in enabling healing. Even "faith healers" ask the patient for a description of his illness and how he understands cure.

The active role of the patient is an important factor in explaining why healing occurs in some cases and not in others. As the patient teaches, she also becomes a healer. These two roles of teacher and healer merge when a patient participates in decisions about her treatment.

A further dimension of the patient as teacher is her ability to teach others about the deepest questions of human existence. Some have even suggested that the act of anointing in the rite of healing could be understood as an anointing for service. People who are sick then can be sanctified to render service to the community through their sickness. They can represent how a person accepts and bears up under illness by reflecting faith, hope, and love. My father reflected these attributes in the last days of his life. He became so weak at age ninety-five that he could not get out of bed, he was eating very little, but he still had a sharp mind. He said to my son, "Though the body is wasting away, the spirit is growing stronger." This testimony to his Christian faith was a powerful witness to us all. The very fact of illness may enhance a person's ability to teach others, to cut to the core of life and set the substantial issues of living into bold relief. Illness galvanizes us to address the most serious questions concerning the purpose of existence, the reason for suffering, the presence of evil, and the nature and existence of God.

The seriously ill person moves away from the superficial and peripheral questions of human existence—"What length dress should I wear?"—and toward a tender appreciation of the wonder of life that may result in the face of catastrophic illness. Based on the image of Jesus Christ as the Suffering Servant, the patient (person), then, in the very state of suffering, becomes a healer, so his strength is in his weakness. The patient's contribution does not depend upon his recovery or his wellness; his illness becomes the basis for his insights. This point does not imply passivity in the face of sickness, but recognizes that healers are not simply those who are free from brokenness; their very brokenness may bring healing to others.

These experiences, growing out of the change from person to patient, enable one to be a teacher by virtue of being a patient. Although Pellegrino recognizes how illness reminds one of the ultimate religious questions, he does not link that to the patient's becoming a teacher. A sick person is forced to confront "last things"—the meaning of illness, death, and God's existence. To be ill is to be reminded of the ultimate fragility of one's personal existence.[35] But his answer to this phenomenon is an additional responsibility for the physician. The physician who hopes to fulfill the obligation to heal, to make the ill patient whole again, must take these religious aspects of illness into account, especially when cure is not possible and care becomes the major responsibility.[36]

Because of their emphasis on the physician's responsibility to enhance the moral agency of the patient, Pellegrino and others lose sight of the way in which a person's illness already may impart a moral sensitivity. Equating moral agency with autonomy minimizes moral responsibility. The patient may assume a moral responsibility to teach the physician and other health care professionals, family, and friends about the deeper values of life through the shared experience of her illness; from this springs compassion, which Pellegrino highlights as the hallmark of the humanistic physician.

Another interesting aspect of the patient's role as teacher is its link with advocacy. As James Lynch, a 1998 graduate of Princeton Theological Seminary, pointed out, persons with AIDS have taught us about courage and resilience, and they have become witnesses and advocates for fair allocation of health care resources and for justice and compassion for all independent of physical illness. The New York City–based organization Gay Men's Health Crisis (GMHC) provides an excellent example of this link between teaching and advocacy and how persons with AIDS in the 1980s challenged the unresponsiveness of a nation to a major health crisis. Thus, occasionally, a patient through illness may develop broader understandings of care and community and serve as an advocate for reform, community development, and community mobilization.

Most physicians and health care professionals acknowledge the patient's crucial role in following health-affirming lifestyles and complying with recommended treatment. However, they are considerably less comfortable with direct patient involvement in choosing and directing treatment. The tragedies chronicled of desperate parents dragging their leukemia-riddled child from one quack to another or the terminally ill adult submitting himself to one untested drug after another give evidence enough of the possible abuses of self-help approaches to medical care. Critics fear that once the patient's role is enhanced, there will be no quality control of health care services because patients will pursue whatever means they desire for health care—legal or illegal. Other critics similarly fear that the holistic health movement may reverse the historical movement in medicine from sects to science.[37] These criticisms are partly justified, but abuse is no justification for disuse. The critics argue partly for greater attention to patient training. Professionals within existing health care disciplines need to develop effective ways of educating patients concerning their appropriate involvement.

In conclusion, the patient is the central but not the primary healer. The patient is central because she initiates the relationship and enlists other healers. However, once involved in a relationship with professional healers, the patient does not serve as the primary healer. She relies on the expertise and knowledge of the professional. Hence the role of the patient as healer is fluid, but the patient should be actively involved as long as possible.

9

The Pastor, Physician, and
Nurse as Healers

Widening the circle of healers creates a related problem. How should we understand the practical working relationship between professionals, volunteers, family, friends, and the patient? What models are available for designing realistic cooperation? Is an interdisciplinary committee the only solution? How inclusive is the definition of professionals who qualify as healers? As mentioned earlier, economists, sociologists, psychologists, politicians, and social workers can all be involved in healing, but their primary focus is not health care delivery.

The patient, physician, nurse, and pastor are the primary coadventurers for health, assisted by family, friends, and associates. However, all are agents of healing. God alone is the source of healing. Physicians, nurses, and pastors are the primary professional healers because their central calling is as health care professionals and they are involved in the two major health care institutions, that is, the hospital and the church. (Here a distinction is in order between those medically and theologically trained and those who within that training have health care as their primary focus. Pastors and chaplains, not theologians, are health care providers in this analysis, and clinical practitioners, not research scientists, are considered health care professionals.) This chapter will examine the pastor, physician, and nurse as individual healers as well as how they relate to one another.

THE PASTOR AS HEALER

Although the patient is the central healer, her role is not a solo one. She works in partnership with family, friends, and professional healers. From the perspective of the church as a health institution, the pastor, as the professional of this institution, is one of the healers.

All pastors will eventually be confronted with the question of what they think of the healing ministry and how they will be involved. If the pastor says that healing miracles were only for Jesus' time and that physical healing is now the domain of medicine, she will then be guilty of perpetuating an ancient dualism.[1]

Modern psychology has taught us that there is always an emotional dimension to illness, and the minister can understand this as the spiritual dimension. What is important to remember is that healing is a part of general ministry. It does not consist only in discrete functions labeled "healing ministries." As the church becomes a therapeutic community, it carries forward Christ's healing ministry. Of course, the more effective the pastor is in general ministry, the more people will seek out the church as a place of healing.

As one who ministers in Christ's name, the pastor is a healer in several ways. First, she is a healer by putting people in touch with the sacramental and devotional resources of the church. The pastor's most important task is to teach people how to pray so that they can experience God as the source of healing. The visitation of the sick is a crucial part of ministry, but it must be more than social chitchat. The laying on of hands should not be viewed as a magic rite promising physical cure, but neither should it be regarded as devoid of power. Leslie Weatherhead suggests that the healing service can be a symbol of the blessing of God and the affirmation that God is with us, no matter what happens. He views the laying on of hands as conveying the "odic force" rather than being a sacramental service.[2] Another basic question is whether the pastor should, in fact, be viewed solely as a healer. Do her prophetic and priestly roles pull her away from the nurturing and counseling relationship to a person? No, they should complement, not compete with, them.[3]

Second, the pastor is a healer as she proclaims the universal truth in the particular situation. These truths include the following: that each person has infinite worth; that illness is not necessarily a sign of sin; that when sin does cause illness, forgiveness is available; that death, though an enemy, has been conquered and need no longer be feared. Furthermore, she can provide a prophetic function calling to mind the spiritual resources and theological truths about health, healing, and healers. Pointing to God's love as reflected in all healing is crucial and may include showing how even medical diagnosis, prognosis, and therapy may have Christological dimensions.[4]

Since the pastor, unlike the physician, does not usually deal in categories of sickness, she is freer to clarify the individual nature of the person's illness. Medical statistics that only one in a hundred is disabled with an illness are little comfort if you are in the 1 percent. The pastor is oriented toward restoration rather than diagnosis, so she can move away from a statistical approach to illness. The pastor is concerned with affirming the person's sense of worth in the face of the limitations and sufferings of illness. This task involves listening as well as speaking.

Third, the pastor conveys the symbols of health and healing, relating to people as persons, not as patients. (One must admit that pastors sometimes label people as sinners to be judged rather than individuals to be helped.) As people face sickness and struggle to regain some wholeness, they are challenged to accept and overcome the undeniable fact of their fragility. Symbols of healing may involve sustenance in the face of pain and suffering—assisting people to live in the midst of their brokenness. The questions emerge: What is the ultimate concern? Where does one stand amidst the ambiguities of suffering? What does one believe about health and disease?

There are three possible answers. The ultimate truth lies in despair and disintegration, and all attempts to use positive healing resources are against our basic nature. From this perspective, there is no sense in struggling against disease because treatment is wrong and to be avoided. This may sound stark, but it is the logical outcome of promoting only the negative side of life. One sees it sometimes in patients who refuse therapy.

On the opposite side is the view that although disease is real, the ultimate truth about the relationship between human nature and disease is that one must struggle against it. This is seen in the natural attempts of the human body to reject disease by its development of antibodies, and in the care and concern of the medical, nursing, and allied health professionals.

The final possibility is a middle-of-the-road, noncommittal path. Here disease and healing are equally important or unimportant. An attitude of indifference prevails.[5] The pastor may help the patient to identify with the symbols of healing, to interpret the symbols, and to cooperate with the physician and the hospital.

The pastor as healer also counsels individuals in order to reveal spiritual roadblocks to healing, to put people in touch with their inner resources for healing, to open them to God's power of healing, and to integrate them into a support and service community, that is, the church. The pastor enters into a covenant relationship not unlike that of the physician. Trustworthiness and constancy are parts of the counseling ministry.

The pastor perhaps more than any other professional must integrate the professional and the personal to be effective in her work. It is of little good to hear a spiritually uplifting message one day, and then to see it vanish in the pastor's personal life and relationships the next day. The pastor's experience of life, suffering, sacrifice, and joy can be the basis for support and sympathy not only during periods of illness and stress, but also during the ordinary life of a person. The pastor, unlike the physician, has the opportunity to develop relationships with her parishioners at times other than crisis and sickness.

The final function of the pastor as healer is to assist the patient in making health care decisions. She should interpret the tradition of the religious community that she represents. Here she functions as a moral expert on the tradition. (Today, very few people adhere completely to a particular creed or denomination, but pick and choose what they like from several traditions. This is seen most clearly in Roman Catholics' practice of abortion. Despite the Catholic Church's teaching against abortion, it happens at the same rate as in the Protestant population.) The pastor in this role can support the decision maker in the midst of all his doubts and anxieties. Many times one's personal views and the church's teachings may conflict; hence the pastor assumes a counseling role to help the person struggle through his choices. One must assist the person to clarify his values, and be a moral guide without being judgmental. Confidentiality is the hallmark of this relationship.

Knowing when and to whom to refer people with needs beyond a pastor's expertise is especially important. Referrals are often part of helping people to make decisions. Linking a person with various health care professionals and community resources can assist in making the right decisions. For example, in death and dying decisions, linking people with the Society for the Right to Die may help them with their decisions. Knowing when and to whom to refer a patient is crucial, whether the referral is to a psychiatrist, psychologist, or thanatologist. This pastoral role, as an assistant in decision making, may be a new and very important role for the church as bioethical quandaries expand.

This discussion of the role of the pastor as healer may appear to idealize rather than describe how pastors function. Appropriately, one needs to ask how a pastor can be equipped to fulfill this role. This is especially true in light of the fact that for many physicians, clergy are viewed as part of the problem rather than bearers of healing. For patients, they may sometimes bring more trouble than comfort, for example, judgment of sin and resultant guilt.

The pastor's tools as a healer are primarily words. Cassell emphasized for physicians the importance of language as a tool in healing; how much more this is true for pastors. A pastor's training is almost entirely in words, touch is infrequent, and medicine and surgery are not available for her use. However, the pastor may need to cultivate more of a ministry of presence—standing by in the face of sickness and suffering when words are inappropriate.

While it is true that the pastor has a crucial role in a healing ministry, recognizing one's limitations is also important. More harm than good can be done, especially in the area of persons with addictions to alcohol/drugs and other forms of substance abuse as well as perpetrators or victims of sexual abuse and domestic violence, by well-meaning clergy. Because there are spiritual and psychological dimensions to these illnesses in addition to physiological and sociological ones, pastors may operate with the illusion that they can treat these cases, causing undue suffering and damage as a result. Building a good referral network may be the most essential contribution a pastor can make as part of the healing team.

The pastor as a healer raises some practical problems. What is her relationship to the secular patient or health care professional? How will her services be reimbursed? Does a sick person have less of a chance for health without the clergy? In response to the last question, the answer is yes if one concedes that spiritual health constitutes part of what is meant by health as wholeness. For example, David Castle suggests that spiritual as well as physical checkups are needed, and we should endeavor to find ways to reenergize the spiritual life. One questionnaire, with sections on beliefs and practice, on personal maturity and ministry, has been designed to help generate a spiritual health inventory.[6] In fact, a number of spiritual assessment instruments are currently being developed. Of course, even the "religious" person is not dependent on the clergy to put him in touch with spiritual resources, but the pastor may encourage and facilitate that to happen.

The problem of compensation has not been resolved. Currently, the third-party payment system and even HMOs rarely cover pastoral counseling. In the Wholistic Health Care Centers, Inc., where the pastor is one of the four or five professionals on the health team, the pastor's services are covered only under the initial health inventory consultation, not in separate counseling sessions. The medical consultation, but not the spiritual consultation, qualifies as health care. In the British National Health Service this seems to be regarded somewhat differently because chaplains are paid under the NHS.

The pastor's relationship to the secular patient should be one of openness. Seemingly nonreligious patients may suddenly become concerned with spiritual questions as a result of their illness or that of a loved one. Being available to respond to those situations is important. We should go where needed without question or judgment. In many cases these people may be friends or relatives of church members or acquaintances who are at their wits' end. The pastor as healer offers many rich opportunities for a ministry to all persons.

THE PHYSICIAN AS HEALER

In a discussion of the role of healers, physicians and nurses are crucial to an integrated approach to healing. There are not several types of healing, that is, medical, spiritual, and mental, but one source of all healing—God. God uses all means to display divine healing power. The discussion here is not about the nature of medicine or even the work of physicians per se, but how they relate to other healers, including the patient.

Behind the question of the physician's relationship to other healers is the determination of the appropriate health problems to which the physician should respond. There are two operative models: complaint and scientific. In the complaint model of medicine the physician responds to all the patient's problems and needs; in the traditional scientific model only problems that can be treated by drug or surgical therapy are accepted.[7]

One of the tensions created by expanding the definition of healers is understanding whether the physician relates to them in a primary or secondary role. On the one extreme are those who view the physician as a general. This perspective was reflected, for example, in the 1983–84 debate over Bill 5-166 in Washington, D.C., regarding the role of alternative health professionals in hospitals, here referring to nurse-midwives, podiatrists, psychologists, nurse practitioners, and nurse anesthetists. In objecting to their access to hospitals, Dennis O'Leary, former president of the D.C. Medical Society, wrote,

> We look forward to working with allied health professionals in and out of hospital settings with the same confidence we have always had in their commitment and competence. We simply ask that the Council [Washington, D.C.] recognize that in the war on disease, as with all other wars, there must by definition be soldiers and generals. There is an absolute need for expert command in the battle against illness. And, for all the triumphs as well as all the heartbreak, it falls to the physician to guide, and to serve with all of his legions in offering comfort.[8]

Others understand the physician as a type of field officer who marshals the resources to confront illness. Pellegrino reflects this view as he describes the doctor who hears all the needs, then parcels them out to the appropriate experts. Cassell envisages the physician as the one who meets many of the patient's needs. Tournier describes the physician as a type of suffering servant figure, carrying all the problems within himself. He even suggests the ordination of doctors as ministers in recognition of their "religious" calling.[9] Tournier continues:

> [The] vocation of medicine is a service to which those are called who through their studies and the natural gifts with which the Creator has endowed them . . . are specially fitted to tend the sick and to heal them. Whether or not they are aware of it, whether or not they are believers, this is from the Christian point of view fundamental that doctors are, by their profession, fellow workers with God . . . because their activity is itself a sign of God's patience.[10]

The prayer of the Christian doctor is not "God, help me," but "God, use me." It is an interesting phenomenon now that the belief of people is not in the church's power to heal but in that of the medical profession. People who possess the gift of healing outside medicine are at best considered eccentric.

However, one must acknowledge that the medical profession itself is going through radical change not only because of managed care but also because of the impact of the Generation X mentality on the meaning of vocation. ("Generation X" is the term used to describe persons born in the United States between 1963 and 1981.) With the advent of an increased number of female doctors, doctors and others are looking for fulfillment outside their jobs in family, friendships, and spirituality.[11] Physicians historically were seen primarily as self-sacrificing. The Declaration of Geneva, for example, gives clear expression to this view: "At the time of being admitted to the medical profession: I solemnly pledge my life to the service of humanity. . . . The health of my patient will be my first consideration."[12]

Pellegrino provides a clear vision of the physician's calling at its best. First, the physician is to restore wholeness; to assist in striking a balance between what the body imposes and the self aspires. The doctor is seen as the healer par excellence. "Only healing requires the physician as physician because its end cannot be achieved by others in society."[13] (This view, of course, is different from the one presented here.) The physician's self-healing may occur while he is healing others, and he often cannot heal others until he himself has been healed. If the patient lacks the skills and knowledge to make himself whole again, the physician must perform that function. "It is to the physician, as a professed healer, that we all turn to assist us in making our humanity whole again—to repair, or reverse the bodily defect and to do so in a way that recognizes the uniqueness of our own experience of illness."[14]

The healing relationship of patient and physician is based on the following: a relationship of trust; the promise of assistance; the forming of a covenant arising out of the vulnerability of the patient; the capabilities of the physician; and an act of profession.[15]

The patient always takes precedence, and the economic well-being of society cannot compete with the urgent need of the patient. When macro and micro health care allocations conflict, only in exceptional circumstances can the interests of the individual patient be set aside.[16] The doctor has the problem of how to limit the resources devoted to a particular patient, which was discussed earlier in relation to managed care.

The personal dimension of the medical encounter is very important; it should be marked not by the transaction of knowledge but by an interpersonal relationship. The objectivity of the physician must be combined with compassion. Medicine without compassion is mere technicism—curing without healing. Even a technically right decision is a value-weighted activity. Knowing the objective prognosis of a particular disease is not enough, since illness is really a subjective experience influenced by the patient's perception of distress. Without compassion, the physician fails to understand both the patient and the illness. The personal interaction between physician and patient is also tied to their belief systems.

A physician may affect the outcome of a therapy by his beliefs. However, the trust of the patient in the doctor is also important. In double-blind placebo tests both the patient's and the doctor's beliefs in the efficiency of the process are crucial. For example, the effectiveness of vitamin E in angina pectoris patients in Jerry Solfvin's research was influenced by the doctor's belief in the medicine. Meprobamate tranquillizer trials also reflected superior results for patients with doctors who believed in its effectiveness. Yet certain drugs work independently of the physician's beliefs because they are so strong or there is a generic belief in them.[17]

Guarding the personal aspect of the patient-physician relationship is difficult against the depersonalizing forces in medicine, that is, the necessity to ground medicine in science, the bureaucratization that places roles over persons, and the commercialization of the profession itself.[18] Physicians should strive for technical knowledge and for virtues that set apart the best doctors. Truth telling, disclosure, promise keeping, assisting in the patient's autonomous decision, helping the patient to cope and adjust to illness are all the roles of physicians. The physician becomes the principal person to organize the treatment of the patient in the face of the often immobilizing effect of illness and to guard the patient's right to define what is the best treatment.[19]

Despite this major emphasis on the personal dimension of medicine and the need for humanistic characteristics in the physician, medicine does not reduce to art. Compassion is no substitute, for example, for surgical incompetence. Competence is absolutely fundamental to the practice of medicine. However, the physician must use all the knowledge of technology for the patient's best interests. "Do no harm" must be supplemented with "Do all things essential." Physicians should be healers, not killers, as in physician-assisted suicide, according to C. Everett Koop, former U.S. surgeon general.

Arising out of these responsibilities are certain obligations that a physician incurs by virtue of the original act of profession when entering the physician-patient relationship. These obligations are specific to a particular patient, and the doctor's claim to knowledge bestows a special obligation to the client/patient who needs that information. The professional possesses a monopoly on this knowledge, which produces an inequality of power. This imbalance of power creates the following special obligations for the physician that reflect the intermingling of the technical and moral dimensions of medicine: (1) to be competent, a minimum requirement for being a physician (this competence must be shaped by the goal of the medical act to be performed, that is, the right and good healing action for a particular patient); and (2) to facilitate the patient's moral agency by remedying the patient's information deficit. The doctor and the patient must feel and know together. A reformulated Golden Rule reflects this: "We should so act that we accord the patient the same opportunity to express or actualize his own view of what he considers worthwhile as we would desire for ourselves."[20]

The word "patient" itself denotes who he is. The Latin root for "patient"— *patior* (to suffer, to bear something)—was first used in the medical sense by Chaucer. The patient then is searching for restoration to wholeness, and the physician promises to assist in that search. "A doctor gazes at his patient and sees himself, joined they are one pilgrim in search of health."[21] The doctor promises compassion, which links her immediately to the patient, since compassion and suffering with a patient have the identical root.

Because the patient suffers an ontological assault, the dimension of anguish in illness separates the patient-physician relationship from that of lawyer-client or teacher-pupil. The patient's vulnerability is sometimes reflected in his inability to heal himself, and in the lack of the necessary knowledge or skills to restore his health; he is part of a wounded humanity. Furthermore, his state of harmony is never the same after illness. In light of this state, the physician makes a promise to heal (make whole)—to use her knowledge, skill, and competence to that end. However, this should be in partnership with the patient. Technical competence is not enough; it should be balanced with compassion. Part of this compassion includes assisting the patient to the extent necessary to make conscious choices; he is not just an object of technical manipulation.

Another aspect of the doctor's work is the use of language. Spoken language provides the physician with a most important tool. The healer must be precise and fully explain a patient's illness and treatment. Patients inevitably interpret silence as a sentence to the worst possible disease. Body language, including eye contact, is also crucial. Feelings generated in the doctor's office should be addressed to assuage a patient's fears.

In Cassell's medical practice, he emphasizes the importance of communication; "conversation" includes listening for what is behind a patient's words. Words are to the general practitioner as scalpels are to the surgeon.[22] In a typical case, a wife has cancer, and her husband imagines that his pinched nerve is really an imminent heart attack because he fears a debilitating condition that would make it impossible for him to care for her. He believes that he has successfully hidden his fears from his wife, but she is already aware of what is happening. All these facts are slowly revealed through a consultation with both of them.

Patient-physician communication is important. Cassell, echoing P. Lain Entralgo, links the Hippocratic tradition to the breakdown in communication between physician and patient for the following reasons: (1) when avoiding the earlier magical chants, physicians also dropped the spoken word as part of their healing ministrations; (2) patients no longer participated in their own healing since diagnosis was based on objective data, which the patients could not furnish, so their perspective did not matter; and (3) disease was objectified.[23] When the spoken word languishes, communication dies.

This trend of objectification should be replaced by a bonding between patient and physician, which enhances the physician as teacher. It is forged to a large extent by words exchanged. Bonding, as well as transference, occurs in the patient-physician relationship where feelings of anxiety and discouragement can flow back and forth between physician and patient. In fact, the sicker the patient, the stronger are these ties since the patient becomes more open and direct.[24] One should note, however, that this happens only if the relationship is already on an honest, open footing; otherwise, there is an avoidance of the deep issues. Natural bonding, conversation, and the laying on of hands may all be part of healing. Hence the physician's connectedness and her omnipotence are important tools for healing. This nurturing, almost maternal role of the physician reminds us of similar descriptions by E. D. Pellegrino and W. F. May. (See especially May's insightful book *The Physician's Covenant: Images of the Healer in Medical Ethics.*) Doctors become both the "patient" and the patient's "agent," forming the basis for physician-patient bonding. This development parallels maternal-infant bonding, though Cassell believes that the physician-patient bond is unique.

One way to determine how the physician relates to other healers is to decide which health problems are his responsibility. Physical medicine does not focus primarily on psychiatric, personal, and lifestyle problems. It is difficult for the physician to motivate the patient toward health or a change of lifestyle patterns. Karl Barth stated, "Can he [the doctor] promote the strength to be as man? No, this is something which each can only will, desire, strive for, but not procure nor attain of himself."[25] When the doctor acknowledges this fact, he is free to help where he can.

How can the doctor help? First, the doctor has a crucial role by removing the obstacles to the patient's will for real health. She can assist in providing a milieu for healing to take place. The first rule of medicine, *primum non nocere,* is an admonition to that effect. She cannot provide life purpose and direction, but she can provide an understanding of how health can contribute to that enterprise. Second, if no remedy for an illness is available, she can at least make it relatively bearable. She can minimize the effects of disease and its complications. An example is the control of pain even when its cause cannot be eradicated. Third, she can continue in a covenant relationship with the patient, a relationship marked by promise keeping, truth telling, trust, and ongoing care.

The more difficult area to assess is the physician's role vis-à-vis the suffering that ill health produces. Good medical practice requires a degree of objectivity and technical efficiency. This pressure for efficiency creates tension with the caring and personal side of medicine. Too often a doctor may cover up his sensitivity behind a scientific attitude. Pellegrino describes a physician's compassion ("to suffer with") as a necessary link to the patient (also the terms are etymologically linked). Indeed, the fact of suffering may provide the original impetus to enter medicine. Tournier remarked, "I think the best doctors are those who cannot bear to see suffering, and who try to bring relief and healing in spite of the limitations of our means and who pursue their vocation in spite of the suffering it imposes on them."[26]

Cassell writes eloquently about the doctor's role in helping the patient to confront suffering and death. By dismissing talk of death, medicine denies a person the use and meaning of his own death. His serenity, dignity, or courage in the face of death is no longer valued. When medicine is reduced to science, treatment of sick persons is often limited to using external things on people rather than calling on their internal resources.

For Cassell, the two priorities of the physician are (1) defense against imminent death and (2) defense against disability. Priority one, now from a medical perspective, is more easily won and still receives the major emphasis. However, imminent death and treatment of acute disease are no longer the greatest problem; rather, dealing with life is where we have the greatest need.[27] Because acute diseases are no longer the major problem, medicine now deals with chronic or disabling illness. In disabled, even terminal patients, symptoms not related to their major disease should also be treated. All too often, nonfatal symptoms of a dying patient are not considered worthy of treatment—for example, back pain in a cancer patient. But that back pain may be the most annoying aspect of being sick.

Contemporary attitudes toward death are ambivalent. It is considered good practice to tell the truth to dying patients; death in a sense has come out of the closet. Yet while there is pressure for technological restraint in the care of the dying, death is still viewed as a failure of technology to rescue the body.

The attempt at a detached or "objective" position toward death circumvents the process of mourning and prevents the physician from having a sensitive involvement with patients.[28] (The physician's attitude can affect the person's ability to cope with dying.) One of the doctor's responsibilities is to grant the patient permission to die. This results from an assessment of what the patient really wants. It is possible, however, that labeling a patient as "dying" may indicate to a patient that the doctor can no longer help.[29] Facing death involves helping the patient to name his fears, such as losing the family, missing a son's wedding, or missing a daughter's graduation. If a dying patient says, "I'm afraid," the physician should press him to name the fear. This is the first step toward dispelling it since fear of the unknown, not the fear of cessation of consciousness, is the primary angst. The physician then is called upon to help the patient remain in control while dying—to teach the patient the best control of pain, the use of his body, and the various things that he can do. Cassell is adamant about the importance and feasibility of relieving pain in the dying patient. There is absolutely no excuse for suffering caused by pain. It may require ingenuity and patience on the part of the physician to prevent such pain, but it is possible.

This extension of the physician's Asclepian authority from bestowing the sick role to granting permission to die seems precariously close to usurping God's authority over life and death. What happens when the physician determines that it is time to die and the patient still wants to battle for life? In Cassell's analysis, this conflict would not occur, since the physician accompanies the patient along the dying process and assesses in light of the entire journey when she is ready to die. Clearly, Cassell's position stems from compassion toward the aged, terminally ill person since he has worked several decades with them. Not surprisingly, he often sees death as a friend, as a welcome relief to the loss of body control, pain, and suffering of the dying process.

Death is a process in which the patient plays a part, and the physician's role in certain cases may be "to actively help the dying patient develop the will to die."[30] The doctor and the patient together acknowledge that the time has come to leave this life. Rather than engendering a feeling of helplessness, this acceptance of death restores dignity and involvement for the patient. The patient can participate in the process of dying, if not death itself.

The innate resistance to death by the patient, as well as those around him, can often border on denial. Physicians can help their patients overcome this denial of death by being honest with them about their condition. Truth telling is a prime virtue for physicians when their patients face death. The medical setting in general and the hospital in particular reinforce passivity, resistance, and denial of death. Of course, with the debates about physician-assisted suicide, the whole doctor-patient relationship vis-à-vis death is changing.

Sometimes the physician can talk frankly only with the patient, not with the family, about his impending death because the family does not want to face it. A family's denial can cause undue suffering to a patient because the doctor is forced to use "extraordinary" measures to keep him alive. Additionally, a conspiracy of silence may loosen the family bonds and create the loneliness of unburdened fears at the very time that the patient most needs his family.

Although Cassell recounts numerous "successful" cases of telling the patient about her impending death coupled with how to remain in control, he warns against a universal policy of "telling all." When denial is the patient's only defense, the physician should support it, that is, treat each case individually. "Patients' right to deny is as basic as their right to be told the truth."[31] However, protecting someone from painful information may increase uncertainty and paralyze action because it conflicts with other information. If the doctor does not discuss her case, the patient concludes she is surely beyond the pale, past any real help, and is subject to her own fears and fantasies about the prognosis of her disease.[32] This does not mean burdening the patient with every detail of a remotely possible illness in order to protect the doctor from a malpractice suit. The care of the dying, as of the living, should take place within, and not override, except in special circumstances and for short periods, the framework of the person's life.

Cassell rightly points out some positive side effects of facing death honestly. In discussing, for example, patients whose burns are so extensive that they cannot survive, he notes two discoveries made by health care teams: (1) the truth of their terminal condition did not fill them with despair; they became quite peaceful; and (2) despite the initial difficulties of dealing honestly with patients, in the end candor is the best policy.[33]

Although Cassell's description of the dignity of a patient welcoming his own death compels, it also disquiets. One of the reasons is his emphasis on the physician's role in the death scenario: "The doctor must openly face his responsibility. He must be right, in the light of his knowledge and judgment, that indeed the time has come for the patient to leave."[34] Cassell continues, "In the case of the dying, based on trust and the service of his patient, the physician can give permission for the person to stop the battle for life."[35] But how would this authority be used by a less compassionate physician? Potential organ donation, need for hospital beds, or burdens on a family could quickly slip in as justifying causes to give permission to die.

Death introduces the transcendent. In one sense, the conversations about death occur outside time because, for the dying patient, successive time may shift into simultaneous time—past, present, and future are all now. Most patients use time-space subjectively, a point to remember when gathering data on a patient. This transcendent dimension raises religious questions surrounding death that Cassell does not address.

According to him, terminally ill patients seldom ask, "Why me?" And if they do, his answer is sometimes things just happen that way. This is to engender not a hands-folded response, however, but a focus on *what* instead of *why*. "You may not make the weather, but you can carry an umbrella."[36]

Cassell concludes that hopelessness results not from having knowledge of impending death, but from feeling abandoned or out of control, or perceiving the doctor as helpless. Hope then is maintained by the degree of autonomy that a patient experiences in his dying. Fear of death is uncommon in dying patients, but wishing to die may be more prevalent. Fear of death may not be the fear of the unknown, but fear of nothingness, separation, and disappearance. Fear for most patients is not of death itself, but of the process of dying—pain, nausea, thirst, and weakness.

Cassell may be correct in arguing that the process of dying holds more fear than the state of death, but questions surface about what happens after death. He does not address the fears that can accompany the physical anguish of bodily pain and discomfort. Is there life after death? Will I continue to exist as a unique individual? Will I see again the people I love—or perhaps worse, those I hate? These "spiritual" questions need to be addressed for dying persons, or their "pain" will not abate simply by learning to control their bodies. It is here the presence of the pastor/priest/rabbi as a member of the health team is so important. This caring response to illness colors the patient-physician relationship. How does viewing the patient as healer influence it? The bonding image that both Pellegrino and Cassell embrace may be too passive a model if the patient is really to become responsible for her own care. Its strength is its focus on people, not diseases. It emphasizes primarily the caring dimension of the relationship, but neglects the educational aspect, which is equally important.

On the other hand, the client and consumer image in a contract model that is usually used to describe the relationship when the patient assumes a more active role is not necessarily desirable.[37] Whatever model is used, revisions in medical education are needed if the patient-physician relationship is to change. The emphasis must shift from disease treatment to disease prevention and health maintenance, and from the disease itself to the ill person.[38] Under the criticisms of the medical model, the inadequacies of current medical education to train practitioners to respond to the full range of health-related needs have been discussed. As our understanding of health, healing, and healers broadens, this will require even more extensive revisions in the philosophies of medical and theological education.

Although studies reveal a new interest by physicians concerning the importance of health maintenance, less than 1 percent of the health dollar is spent on health education.[39] Most physicians agree with the surgeon general's recommendations regarding the importance of eliminating smoking, moderating caloric intake, and using seat belts in promoting health. Considerably less agreement, however, exists about other health-contributing factors such as exercise, moderate alcohol use, and nutrition.[40]

THE NURSE AS HEALER

Much of what has been written about the physician as healer applies to the nurse since modern nursing and medicine have traveled similar but unequal roads in their approach to caring for people who are sick. The religious "calling" to nursing as a profession is still viewed by many to be essential. Indeed, the struggle to get comparable pay for comparable work continues to be hampered by the ideal of nursing as a religious calling that provides "greater rewards," a view harbored by legislators, health care administrators, and some nurses. The often cited dichotomy that the physician cures while the nurse cares may reflect the different emphases in their respective education but not the reality that the practice of curing and caring should be the business of both professions.

Since the time of caring for the wounded in the Crimean War, nurses have been at the forefront of compassionate care. That was vividly seen in a World War II story told by Ruth Zerner, professor of history at Lehman College in the Bronx, New York.

In Berlin, fifty-five years ago, my aunt was a thirty-two-year-old registered nurse living and working in the bucolic, sprawling campus of a Lutheran hospital, old age home and conference center called *Johannesstift* (*House of St. John*). "Creative survival" describes how nurses in this place of healing responded to the crises connected with Adolf Hitler's war, started in September 1939, when Nazi Germany invaded Poland and when Hitler ordered the systematic killing of mentally ill and physically handicapped persons, those deemed, in the dictator's words, "useless eaters."

According to my aunt's account, the supervising nurse of the Christian residence for senior citizens devised a way to save her senile patients. The Nazis did not order nurses in private, Christian institutions to kill their patients by lethal injection. *That* order was issued by doctors and carried out by nurses in the state-run hospitals and homes. Nazi governmental officials, however, prepared "hit lists" of senile patients who were to be transferred from private institutions to state hospitals. Recognizing that these persons were destined for death, the supervising nurse at my aunt's hospital secretly struck a deal with her counterpart at the state hospital: senile patients were to be transferred on paper, but not in reality. The bureaucratic record indicated that the patients had been removed and extinguished, but Lutheran nurses in *Johannesstift* had surreptitiously found private homes for their targeted seniors, usually with patients' family members or with humanitarian rescuers, who illegally bought ration coupons to feed these helpless elderly persons who were officially dead.[41]

There are still courageous and compassionate nurses, but by and large the nursing profession itself has radically changed. Part of the struggle in nursing has been between caring and power. Because the nursing profession is predominantly female, women's general discomfort with power is further exacerbated by the male-dominant physician world.[42] In prevailing patriarchal ideologies power and caring are posited as polar opposites whereas in new paradigms that need not be the case. New movements refer to empowered caring.[43]

Some scholars have taken a rather dim view of the position of nurses, likening them to the crew who know their place vis-à-vis the captain physician[44] or the submissive wife to the dominant husband. Furthermore, these scholars conclude that the patient is seen by both as a child.[45] These images seem a bit archaic or exaggerated, but it must be admitted they still reflect a kernel of truth. Curing has always rated higher than caring and is more in line with the interventionist medical model. As well, active curing is seen as more masculine while passive caring is viewed as more feminine.

In the United Kingdom, some believe that the current predicament of nursing is that it is a woman's occupation in a man's world, which is marginalized both by medicine and by the British government. The irony is that now politicians and economists who are undermining doctors may add a new dimension to the interface of medicine and nursing. In the United Kingdom, there is discussion of nurses assuming some of the traditional functions of doctors, perhaps to the enrichment of both.[46] In addition, nursing theorists have challenged the medical model's view of care and the morals that have underpinned health care professions. Nurses are now taught to be autonomous practitioners who replace patient care with case management and psychological and emotional counseling techniques. So contemporary nursing, too, seems to suffer from the cult of autonomy. Many are afraid as a result that the founding values of compassionate care in the National Health Service will be lost.[47]

There are other shifts in nursing due to the change from infectious diseases to chronic illness. In response to the changing health needs of the population that have resulted from the aging of the society, nurses are focusing on health promotion both within and outside the institutional setting. Increasingly, the nurse's healing role is in the promotion of self-care and health regardless of the health state. Nurses recognize that health is defined by the individual and that one may have a terminal illness but define his overall health as good from a wholistic perspective; people are more than their bodies. Too frequently the provision of these services is based on economics. Who pays for services such as health education, lifestyle modification programs, self-help groups, assessment and screening, self-care promotion, health counseling for individuals and families, resource and referral services, and alternative therapies such as prayer, meditation, and therapeutic touch?

Discharge planning is a growing area of nursing responsibility. (Parenthetically, here the church can become involved with support services for the homebound, recently released hospital patient.) Nurses with advanced preparation are providing care in more autonomous settings in the community and in long-term care settings. They are serving as the primary healers, as case managers, and as integrators of health care for individuals, families, and communities.

Changes in Nursing in the Wake of Managed Care

The future of nursing is being shaped more by outside forces than by changes within the profession. During the 1980s, nursing schools were pressured to boost enrollment. Now, pressures to reduce inpatient hospital care means fewer acute care beds in hospitals and fewer nurses needed. With hospitals downsizing, the overall vacancy rate was about 4 percent in 1994, down from 17 percent in 1990. There is now a shift of nursing jobs from inpatient care to outpatient and home care. However, out of nearly 1.9 million employed registered nurses, two out of three still work in hospitals. Of nurses surveyed, more than three-quarters said they believed the quality of patient care had been degraded as a result of the cutbacks in staff nurses. Nurses move from crisis to crisis unable to anticipate overall patient needs.[48]

If physician-assisted suicide becomes the norm, one may no longer need the nurse who supports dying persons through their pain and suffering. If cost containment is the greatest virtue, then the caring function recedes into the background.[49] In the 1990s, especially with managed care, one saw the shift from hospital to community-based and ambulatory care settings, including homes, neighborhood clinics, and wellness centers. The nurse, much like the doctor before her, is moving further and further away from patient care to case management. With the advent of all the nurse extender models, the registered nurse (RN) now assumes the role of supervisor, delegator, and trainer.[50] She no longer performs basic functions of bathing and taking temperatures and blood pressures that provided the basis for understanding the patient.

Much of the difficulty of nurses to shape their future stems from their history as helpers rather than leaders in the health care hierarchy. Since the founding of modern nursing by Florence Nightingale, a nurse's image was that of a ministering angel of mercy and the doctor's assistant. Technological medicine was first seen as the purview of doctors with nurses in the auxiliary or secondary role of caring for the patient whose treatment plan was developed outside their authority.

It is not surprising that the advent of managed care has affected the nursing profession as much as, if not more than, other health care professions. Numerous articles in the 1990s highlighted how commerce rather than caregiving became the rule of the day as nursing staffs in hospitals were reduced in large numbers.[51]

Complementary Models in Nursing

In addition to cutting the number of nurses, in many settings they have been replaced by unlicensed personnel and undertrained nurses' assistants. Staff mix models began in the United States in the 1980s as a result of the nursing shortage and then later as cost savings measures.[52] The role of the nurse extender since then has been expanding. The purpose of these models was to free the nurse for patient care while the extenders did housekeeping and stocking of supplies. However, in some instances they have replaced the nurse, which has led to dissatisfaction with these new patterns. A number of complementary models are in place.[53]

The staff mix models used in nursing are of two varieties, that is, *complementary* models (in which support staff who are unlicensed workers do non-nursing work), or *substitution* models (in which some nursing functions are performed). There may be blends between these two models. This is combined with multiskilling, where staff develop new knowledge and skills not originally a part of their specialty but because of downsizing have been forced to take on new responsibilities. The nurse extender model with a nurse assistant or other extender positions actually decreased patient care time because the patient ratio shifted from 1:4 to 1:7.[54]

A 1991 report of the American Hospital Association identified that 97 percent of its member hospitals used some type of nurse extender.[55] The vocabulary used to describe these nurse extenders is constantly expanding. Patient care specialty technicians (PCSTs) are assuming more and more of what was thought of as the central role of RNs. This model in an intensive care unit in Texas is projected to save $1 million.[56] In a study conducted by Pearson and Schwartz in 1990 in an Illinois hospital, using certified nursing assistants and nurses resulted in a 50 percent decrease in the number of RNs employed and $832,688 saved in less than a year.[57]

Preliminary studies seem to suggest that neither patient satisfaction nor quality of care is adversely affected by these new models, but some are concerned that these conclusions are premature.[58] The Manthey "partners in practice" model seems to have been fairly successful with the nurse making the decisions and the technical assistant doing the work; they are able to do the work of two nurses at considerably less expense.

The Twenty-First-Century Nurse

In addition to these emerging models, the RN's job is changing dramatically. On the one hand, the nurse may be moving toward a more powerful position. An original goal of nursing was to be responsible for public health, but that was never realized. One could say, however, that nurses came into their own with the Nursing Agenda for Health Care Reform in June 1991. It presented a core benefits package based on a community health model that emphasized patient self-determination and prevention, and not just sickness care. As well, nurses are becoming autonomous health care practitioners caring for patients in the home with nurse-centered consultation models.[59]

Nurses are now the fourth largest health care political action committee in the United States.[60]

The nurse may have more autonomy, but some question whether the raison d'être of nursing is under fire. The twenty-first-century nurse executive must be able to codify nursing practice according to emerging technologies, to articulate nursing outcomes in cost effectiveness and patient satisfaction, and to extend patient care to "cyberspace" case management and collaborative communities. Nursing as a business unit somehow jolts the common conceptualization of nursing.[61]

Due to changes in health care, the computerized patient record is a necessity for nurses and tends to make wholistic care difficult because of atomic reporting necessities.[62] It is possible that as experience working with taxonomies grows, they can be wholistic rather than atomistic, but that is not necessarily easy.

As nursing has moved closer to a scientific model, it has sometimes considered the more subjective categories of spirituality and spiritual needs as inappropriate. Surveys have shown that the majority of nurses fail to do spiritual assessments or even pray or discuss spiritual concerns with their patients.[63] The suggestion here is not, however, that all nurses have lost their wholistic skills and have become depersonalized administrators.

Nurses are still educated in the wholistic concept of persons and the art and science of meeting human needs whether they are physical (disease), psychological (self-esteem), sociological (relationships), or spiritual (meaning in life). The application of the wholistic concept of human nature, which was discussed earlier, is demonstrated in nursing practice by the wholistic health assessment of the individual, family, or community; respect for autonomy in health care decision making; promotion of self-care abilities; intervention to compensate for a deficit in self-care; and advocacy for social and environmental changes to facilitate health and healing.

Nurse scholars such as Virginia Henderson, Martha Rogers, and more recently Ruth Stoll and Norma Small have affirmed that a wholistic approach requires attention to the spiritual dimension. In the late 1990s, the spiritual dimension of patient care began to return in nursing as evidenced by the design of spiritual assessment instruments and the expansion of the parish nurse subspecialty. Spirituality is most often defined as being in touch with the transcendent. It also involves a sense of well-being in relation to God, belief in a purpose to life, and hope for the greater goals of life here and forever. It is distinct from religion and religious practices, which are a subset of one's spirituality.[64] Constance Sumner, an oncology nurse at Allegheny University Hospital Medical College of Pennsylvania, is representative of that trend. She and others have described spiritual distress in patients and use a "spiritual needs protocol," which outlines assessment, interventions, reportable conditions, and documentation.[65]

Organizations such as the American Holistic Nurses Association (AHNA), founded about twenty years ago, help to highlight the importance of an integrated care model. The goal of its members is to work to free the patient's physical, emotional, and spiritual energy. The best-known modalities used are therapeutic touch, biofeedback, guided imaging, hypnotherapy, meditation and prayer, music, and art.[66]

The nurse's preparation in assessing spiritual needs (spiritual distress is an accepted nursing diagnosis) enables her to respond to symptoms within the context of her nursing practice. It is the nurse who recognizes the need for the professional spiritual advisor and places the call to the pastor or church. It is the nurse who is available to communicate with the pastor or church visitors when they visit in the institution. The nurse has always viewed the pastor as an essential member of the health care team.

The nurse is the best-prepared health care professional, by historical foundations, educational preparation, theoretical base, and practice orientation, to assist the patient in assuming an active role in her own health and, when she has deficits in self-care abilities, to assume the role of integrating the healing resources for the patient. The nurse, then, may provide a link between patient, physician, and pastor. The pastor is viewed not simply as a doctor for the soul but as the bearer of the symbols of hope and healing. She may help people to face and overcome sickness in all its forms. The physician as the medical expert par excellence can cure and empower the patient as well as wage the war against disease. The nurse, by emphasizing patient care as well as advocating for better home health care and patient education, can return the patient to his or her rightful central role. The distinctive contribution of each health care professional has been clarified and the patient's central role affirmed. This leads in the next chapter to the advocacy of a collaborative model, in which the experience and training of the primary health care specialist are maximized and the centrality of the patient is affirmed.

10

The Collaboration of Healers

Now that we have discussed the pastor's, physician's, and nurse's roles, the question arises, How can they cooperate with one another? This book attempts to synthesize the caring role of the health care professionals in society for the care of the sick, ill, or sorrowing patient and her family. In particular, their complementary responsibilities are important. True cooperation between religion, medicine, and nursing depends upon mutual respect. It also requires a recognition that caring and curing are both parts of a response to the patient.

Pastor and Physician as Partners

If, in fact, many persons contribute to our health, it would seem reasonable to incorporate as coequals and collaborators the roles of the pastor, physician, and nurse. The physician-pastor cooperation is our principal focus since there is little written about three-way cooperation or collaboration between the pastor and nurse. There will be a brief mention of the new subspecialty of parish nursing, which since the 1980s has provided new models of cooperation. (This specialty of nursing will be discussed in more detail in my companion volume.) Historically, cooperation between the pastor and the physician was often inhibited by the pastor's belief that sickness originated in sin and the doctor's fear of what this belief would do to the patient. Furthermore, when the sacrament of healing became extreme unction after the twelfth century, the very appearance of the priest might appear to hasten death since the patient anticipated the last rites. (Since Vatican II, there has been a return to the sacrament's original nomenclature: the sacrament of healing.) This was compounded by the heresy that God sends disease, so it is a cross to be borne. This erroneous doctrine of vicarious suffering, as Evelyn Frost names it, is the wolf in sheep's clothing. So the sufferer is pointed to the pains of the cross instead of the joys of the resurrection.[1] The incarnation, not the cross, should form the essential character of the regenerate life.

A thinker who can provide a theoretical basis for the dialogue between medicine and religion, physician and pastor, is Edmund D. Pellegrino. As a devout Roman Catholic layman, a practicing physician with more than forty-five years' experience, and an author of numerous writings on the subject, he is one of the best representatives of the physician's viewpoint.

Pellegrino's views on the relationship between the disciplines of religion and medicine frame his perspective on the spiritual resources for health services. He values these resources and agrees that they have been neglected. Essentially, he views medicine and religion as two separate and distinct disciplines. Even as a practicing Roman Catholic, he does not regard theology as the queen of the sciences, or even a lady-in-waiting.[2] However, he grants theology equal or superior status to philosophy, in contrast to most bioethicists who "leave God in the hall" as a requirement to enter the classroom of medical ethics dialogue. Pellegrino accepts both science and theology as important health resources, but science remains the organizing discipline for health care. "Medicine as a disciplined body of knowledge is a science respecting the perfection of lived bodies concretized by skill in experiencing and effecting connections between corporeal symptoms and remedies."[3]

Religion heals with words; medicine heals the body directly. (Contrast this with Cassell's view that language is a tool of medicine.) Even though the moral may touch on the physical with its healing power, Pellegrino draws a sharp distinction between medicine and religion. Medicine deals with diseases through symptoms and organic causes; religion deals with expressions of bodily disorder. Religion then works on the lived self through the body by action-at-a-distance, that is, words. Medicine works directly with the body. Hence medical judgment is distinct from moral judgment because medicine is concerned with a lived body and psychiatry and religion with the lived self.[4]

Although Pellegrino's aim is to show the proper sphere of each discipline, his sharp distinction between religion and medicine invites dualism. Sharply separating these lines bifurcates body and spirit. Some would argue that the interaction of body, mind, and spirit in a sick person is observable both in the doctor's office and in the pastor's study. What of the healing effect of the doctor's presence when he is just "standing by," as Lewis Thomas expressed it? Or the physical cures that have resulted with the priest's administration of the sacrament of healing or the laying on of hands? Furthermore, these two religious acts involve contact with the patient's body, blurring this sharp division of spheres. The nurse may offer an effective bridge between the physician and the pastor by helping to empower the patient and interpret her needs when necessary.

Despite his attempts to retain separate spheres of operation for religion and medicine, Pellegrino acknowledges that religion enriches medicine by more fully recovering the sources of medicine's morality and by enhancing medicine's healing relationship with those it seeks to serve.[5] In relation to the first point, religion provides three ways for grounding medical ethics, which even philosophy cannot give: (1) an ultimate justification for morality; (2) an integral humanism that is the benchmark for judging competing moral concepts; and (3) a call to sublime sacrifice surpassing what philosophers would think "reasonable."[6]

Religion is a needed source of healing if medicine is to mobilize every resource on the patient's behalf. Using the religious resources of healing is crucial to the physician's covenant to help the patient become "whole" again. These resources are especially needed in the case of serious illness where "we must reassemble our whole life and repair our whole humanity."[7] These needs can only be met partially by medication, surgery, and even compassion and caring. Pellegrino observes, "Acknowledgment of God as the source of healing is a needed antidote to the *hubris* that is so seductive to contemporary medicine."[8] And he adds, "There is in every serious illness an encounter with the question of God."[9] Besides assisting the physician, religion may offer the believer the only satisfactory meaning for his illness, suffering, and death.

Pellegrino is not suggesting that religion always is a source of healing and comfort, but for those who believe in God, it may be. Since the religious dimension is so common to humankind, even the nonbelieving physician must take it into account. Because illness raises the ultimate questions for many patients, it is important for the physician to understand something of a patient's belief and value system and how it can be a source of guilt or healing in the patient's life. To repair the wound in one's humanity that is illness, the most significant element is the stance taken in respect to the power beyond oneself. Belief in God requires asking for God's help. For the nonbeliever, this belief in God may be substituted by a stoicism or raging against fate.[10]

Moving from the contrast and cooperation between the two disciplines, Pellegrino addresses the relationship between their healers, that is, pastor and physician. One meeting ground for these two professionals is their mutual interest in people's nature. The philosophical and theological conceptions of humankind have a profound influence on medicine.[11] Metaphysics and the ontology of man/woman are proper concerns for medicine, which has tended to be too exclusively normative in its perspective.[12] Reductionistic biology has caused a neglect of our physiological, psychological, cultural, and social responses.[13] A new synthesis should be forged between philosophy and medicine to overcome our ontological anxiety. The theologian-philosopher can contribute to the physician a broader understanding of human nature. The physician should be interested in human nature and existence since disease is a disorganization of the patient's whole world. In fact, the vulnerability, powerlessness, and inequality of both the sinner and the patient give rise to similar moral obligations for the pastor and the physician but do not imply a correlation between them.[14] In addition, the nurse by training is well suited to foster an understanding between the physician and the pastor as her more wholistic orientation reinforces the need for cooperation between the disciplines.

How are these similar obligations reflected in their healing ministry? First, Pellegrino understands both pastor and physician as responding to a type of religious calling: "Indeed, I would hold that the very highest levels of obligation to the sick are always in some sense religiously inspired."[15] Second, in relation to others, a physician has the primary responsibility for healing. The relationships between the patient, his family, friends, and pastor are important, but the healing element in these relationships is not the central one as it is in medicine. They function as healers temporarily, but this role is not the sole reason for their relationship. They are bound by moral obligations to the patient, but their function is different from that of the physician's.[16] "We would not hold that friends, family, or ministers are practicing medicine. Though they may cooperate importantly in helping the patient's healings they are not required to fulfill the demands of the act of medicine as we have outlined them."[17] (Of course, the fact that other tasks are not classified as medical ones in relation to the patient does not mean they cannot be healing acts.)

Even though Pellegrino considers the physician the primary healer, he recognizes the importance of the minister; it is simply that their tasks are different. Both physician and minister, starting from different ends of the spectrum, confront wounded humanity. Physicians start with the anatomical, physiological, and diagnostic. Ministers begin with the need for reconciliation, dealing with guilt, the meaning of illness, and the person's spiritual destiny. Ministers are involved in the healing of spirit, soul, and psyche. "The minister is the indispensable mediator, with the transcendent power outside man, with whom reconciliation must be effected."[18] The physician works with manipulation, drugs, or reassurance; the minister works with prayer, sacraments, and the preaching of the Word. Both use touch, words of reassurance, and their own presence—that is, standing by the bedside, summoned by the patient's need. Their functions may overlap in the personal, social, and psychological areas of the patient's life. "While he (the physician) should not substitute for the minister or the theologian, he may have to provide medical assistance in the direction of conscience [*Seelsorgehilfe*, one who helps in the care of the soul] as Niedermeyer has suggested."[19]

There is a question whether these clear-cut distinctions of function for the minister and the physician can be maintained. First, such distinctions may perpetuate a dualism—religion for the soul and medicine for the body—which divides the professionals as well as the patient. Although Pellegrino begins by making this division, it blurs as he discusses how these two professionals serve a person's needs. Only *in extremis* are the functions separate, but they meet at the center in the patient's need. The physician and the pastor overlap in the personal experience of a particular patient: "Initially priest and physician meet at the center, in the personal, psychological experience of this patient with his illness. At the center, the dilemma of a unique person, facing a unique experience, priest and physician overlap."[20]

The physician and the pastor may contact the patient at the same point. When a pastor visits a person in the hospital, the pastor is there because of a bodily condition. (Psychiatric illness is excluded for the purpose of this discussion.) Once the pastor is in the patient's room, spiritual questions may emerge, but they did not initially bring the pastor to the hospital. In other words, when the family of a patient call a pastor, they do not generally say, "Come and see Aunt Sophie; she has deep spiritual questions." Rather, they say, "Come and see Aunt Sophie; she's sick."

So, in one sense, the pastor's initial visit is in response to a physical problem that may have spiritual dimensions. In some pastoral visits, "spiritual" questions are never discussed. Of course, in the daily work of a pastor there may be endless visits where no disease is present, but a need for reconciliation or forgiveness is the occasion for the call. However, the sick person's physical condition summons both pastor and physician to his presence.

Pellegrino's general comments about the interface of medicine and religion, physician and pastor, are particularized for the Christian physician. It is here one observes most clearly his strong Roman Catholic roots. The Christian physician must draw his code from revelation and the church's teaching, and go beyond the secular ideals of competence and compassion. He is to mediate Christian values in his healing and counseling relationship. Exhibiting Christlike behavior is more important than marshaling clear principles for ethical decision making. To a large degree this involves helping the patient to understand the spiritual meaning of sickness and suffering, as well as holding respect for the total life of the patient.

To respect the life of others is to respect their relationship with God; this may include charity and tolerance toward those one believes are making the morally wrong decision. The Christian physician should help the patient to draw on her spiritual resources, wrenching from the crisis of illness, the death of a loved one, or the agony of choosing between two evils the meaning of these experiences in God's providence.[21] The Christian physician is called to employ faith informed by reason as together they confront the patient's sickness and suffering.

The Christian physician also sees medicine's obligations to society in a different light. "Quality of life," genetic purity, and cost-benefit analysis are not suitable criteria for health policy decisions. The Christian should unabashedly acknowledge the religious foundations for the value of human

life as they impinge on decisions concerning abortion, euthanasia, or treatment of persons with disabilities.[22] Pellegrino, however, warns us against
abandoning technology as an act of faith. Rather, a Christian worldview
should redeem, not displace, science and its achievements.

The Christian physician's relation to the pastor is somewhat different
from that of the secular physician's. The sharp dichotomy between the two
professionals is gone. Pellegrino encourages familiarity with each other's language and methods, as well as a sharing of responsibilities. "In fact, if each
is to achieve the full potential of his own healing ministry, he will at times
legitimately play some part of the other's role."[23] In this exchange of roles,
the physician begins to view her work as a ministry, and the pastor may
become part of the physician's world as he leaves the pulpit for the hospital
room. To summarize, Pellegrino emphasizes the importance of spiritual
resources for health care, but allows a modified dichotomy between medicine and religion by assigning them separate spheres and tools for healing.

Moving from the perspective of the individual pastor-physician cooperation, one can examine this from the religion-medicine connection in general.
According to Maddocks, the polarization between medicine and the church
can be traced to the twelfth century when the various Lateran Councils of
1123, 1139, and 1163 prohibited monks from studying medicine or church-
men from practicing surgery. The dissection of the human body was declared
sacrilegious. The process of polarization was sealed by the decree in 1566
obligating physicians to enforce penance on the sick.[24]

In these past decades, clergy have been generally subordinated within the
health field. In the 1960s and 1970s in the United Kingdom, there was the
establishment of clergy-doctor associations such as the Institute of Religion
and Medicine. In the United States, the Society for Health and Human
Values was started by Pellegrino and Ron McNeur, a Presbyterian clergy educator. Robert Lambourne, Michael Wilson, and Michael Melinsky provided
a rationale and model for cooperation between mainstream Christianity and
modern scientific medicine.

These cooperative endeavors, however, radically declined from the mid-
seventies to the early eighties. For example, the membership of the Institute
of Religion and Medicine declined 50 percent from 1971 to 1983 and in
1995 was subsumed under the Churches' Council for Health and Healing
(CCHH). This organization in the United Kingdom is providing a model
for more constructive dialogue between clergy and physicians, hence fulfilling renowned British clergyman William Temple's original vision. According
to Pattison, British clergy on the whole find little interest among doctors in
working cooperatively. One reason may be that the early groups were basically white, male, Protestant liberals, and local clergy still operated within
the more conservative sacramental and spiritual models.

The charismatic healing movement has tended to widen the gap between the two professions. In some instances, there has also been a deprofessionalization of church leaders while medical practitioners have become more highly trained. Formerly, religion and medicine were thought to be engaged in a mutual struggle, but now the medical model is being challenged on all sides. Illich and others have exposed the "iatrogenesis," claiming doctors may cause more harm than good. Even avoiding extremists such as Illich, there are numerous critics of the medical model that make clergy wary of work with physicians. Groups such as the Christian Medical Society have brought together doctors sympathetic to the church, but they operate from a medical mission perspective. Yet what is advocated here is somewhat different. One-on-one cooperation between doctors and clergy with the doctor defining the discourse is not enough. Instead, clergy must take a lead role in defining the discussion and the goals and objectives of health care itself, including a radical transformation of the health care delivery system.[25]

Strides were made in England, especially in this century, when the British Medical Association in 1947 stated that qualified medical practitioners and all who have concern for the religious needs of their patients should work together. However, many felt that this statement had little impact on secular medicine, where scientific information has become the end rather than the means to healing. In the United States, things are even worse; the American Medical Association has not even made such statements about cooperation.

Naturally, the ways that this cooperation happens will vary depending on the perspectives and inclinations of both the physician and the pastor, as well as the desires and interests of the patients, their families, and the particular communities. What is possible in a small, integrated community of families who know one another, who have established relationships in an area, and who have a continuing relationship with both professionals will of necessity be of a different nature from those in a large, urban community where there is only transitory, superficial contact among all parties concerned.

It is difficult for doctors and pastors to cooperate if they do not share the same basic values and convictions. More training is necessary so that they can learn about each other's disciplines. There are some who say that Sigmund Freud, even with his radical critique of religion in his discovery of the unconscious mind, opened the way for cooperation between the doctor and the pastor. Another basis for cooperation comes from the philosophical recognition, after the controversies of the eighteenth and nineteenth centuries, that humans are body-mind, a living dynamic. As well, sociology has emphasized that persons belong to a community, so understanding our environment and relationship to other people is part of understanding who we are.

Despite these realities, problems about cooperation persist. The results of a questionnaire sent to Methodist ministers in the industrial area of Durham County, England, is instructive. Although 75 percent of the clergy said in principle they would consult with a doctor on a case, the average number of consults was only four cases in nine years.[26] The reasons offered for the small number were pressures of work, agnosticism of the doctors, lack of knowledge and training on the part of ministers, and professional isolation.[27] One way to foster cooperation is to identify common problems. For example, in the field of alcohol/drug prevention major strides have been made between the two fields in cooperative programs.

The basis for cooperation between pastor and physician is that both are agents of God, who is the source of all healing; both their respective disciplines provide health resources. As Pellegrino points out, religion not only helps ground and refine medical moral philosophy, it also provides a source for authentic healing and, therefore, for the moral conduct of the patient-physician relationship. This view contrasts markedly with Cassell's description of the clergyman as offering a comforting exit, while the physician offers a chance to return to life.

It is unfortunate that a faith-science dichotomy and a mind-body dualism mark our age, which makes physician-pastor cooperation difficult. Physicians need to appreciate spiritual resources in health care, and pastors must learn how to translate these resources into meaningful language and hard data.

The common meeting ground of medicine and theology is the service and love of humankind. To love means to conform one's actions to the concrete needs of one's neighbor. More specifically, the aim of both medicine and theology is to understand more clearly the reason for human suffering and to seek ways to relieve it. As medicine is called upon to sustain life, theology can assist in exploring the meaning of life. Physicians can give the diagnosis for which pastors are not equipped. Pastors can give the support of a caring community to sustain and to help in healing. Especially when no cure is possible, they can reduce suffering, relieve anxiety, and give inner peace during times of stress. When the physician can do no more to heal the ill person, the task of caring for the patient is not over. The patient constantly struggles to adapt. He must not only bear life, but also grow in the face of personal problems. When confronting suffering, the pastor and the physician acutely need each other's support. They are dealing not with a disembodied illness, but a suffering person. Both the doctor, who is faced with an incurable illness despite all efforts at healing, and the pastor, who earnestly prays for healing, are equally in need of God's grace.

In the moments of crisis and failure the pastor may have a special responsibility to sustain the physician. These occasions may range from frequently affirming the importance of the doctor's calling; to wrestling over an ethical dilemma (for example, when a doctor's colleague performs an incorrect procedure in the operating room, does he report her if she will subsequently lose her license?); to assisting doctors in their constant confrontation with old age, disease, and death; to comforting the doctor in the death of a patient when his knowledge was insufficient or he had not done everything possible to save the patient. The pastor needs an enlightened and sensitive concern to these various issues facing the physician. Of course, caring may also be a concern of the physician, as Cassell has so eloquently argued in *The Healer's Art*.

Like other adversities such as war, injustice, and poverty, disease confronts the individual and the community with a call from God to respond to it. It is precisely at the point of crisis and human suffering that the pastor and the physician intersect in responding to the patient's needs. Together these professionals should help the patient to be involved in his own health care. The pastor may lay open the needs of the patient and provide the impetus for him to seek medical treatment, or the physician may be alerted to spiritual questions that are best handled by the pastor. Practically speaking, this entails consultation between the professionals, probably at the initiative of the pastor.

In the relationship between the physician and the pastor, one has a choice between assigning each a separate sphere of healing or developing a collaborative model. In the former model, the pastor would deal with the spiritual and mental problems—the soul, not the body. The physician would care for the body and the mind as it affected the body. In this paradigm the intersection of the clergy and the doctor would be in the area of mental health and counseling. This model perpetuates a division between mind/body/spirit and forces doctors to be body mechanics. If the overlap between these professionals is only at the center, as Pellegrino expressed it, then what happens at the fringes? Pastors are not simply to sustain patients in the midst of illness or provide a comforting exit from life, but help them to return to health. Pellegrino, like others, builds a crisis- or problem-centered cooperative model instead of health promotion as the goal that joins these professions.

Whole-person medicine may open the way for specific cooperation between physicians and clergy. A dramatic example of this at work was the counseling of pregnant teenagers in the Community of Caring project in Baltimore, Maryland. A group of Muslim, Jewish, Catholic, and Protestant clergy along with Robert Coles, a child psychoanalyst, and several health care professionals developed a values-centered pregnancy-prevention curriculum for teens. When this curriculum was used, the unwanted pregnancy rate among black Baltimore teenagers was reduced by 80 percent in the first year.[28]

As important as collaboration is in special projects, there needs to be an ongoing team relationship between doctor and pastor. In a team situation there should be continual referral and consultation. William J. Kimber, author of *The Healing Church*, has suggested a four-way scheme of treatment for pastor and physician cooperation.[29] First, there is the initial approach that provides the medical diagnosis and pastoral visit. Second, there is the period of preparation that includes treatment, confession, and instruction. Third, there occurs the process of healing through medical treatment and the healing rites of the church. Fourth, after the cure, rehabilitation, worship, and community support take place. It is here that one should add the involvement of the nurse who helps to carry out the treatment. A fifth way of clergy-pastor cooperation should be added in the face of an incurable condition. When cure is not possible, the doctor can minimize the side effects and pain of the disease, and the pastor can share the knowledge of God's sustaining power and love. Unfortunately, many pastors feel apologetic about their role as healers rather than seeking ways to develop a cooperative healing ministry with physicians and nurses.

Several questions emerge about this cooperative model. First, how does one adjudicate conflicts between the pastor and the physician concerning what constitutes the best care for the patient? For example, consider a Jehovah's Witness patient whose doctor recommends a blood transfusion, but whose pastor opposes one. A check against this may be Pellegrino's paradigm for a physician's resolution of conflict. This paradigm consists of (1) loyalty to the patient's best interests; (2) application of the ethical principles in light of the principle of beneficence; and (3) assertion of one's own moral agency. However, the solution to conflicts between the two professionals should rest primarily with the patient. This role applies only to the adult, autonomous patient. What of those at the edges of life—the newborn or the elderly comatose? Are their wishes important only if they are valued by someone else, a social person in Engelhardt's terms, or if they meet Joseph Fletcher's twenty criteria for humanhood? The guide should be what the patient would want if able to express herself, not what one would wish if one were the patient. Here again one sees the nurse as the patient advocate who may know the patient better than the doctor, though this is changing rapidly with the use of nurse extenders and rotating shifts where a nursing staff rather than one or two nurses cares for a patient.

The second question is, Who has the primary responsibility for the care of the patient? In one sense, the very question implies a hierarchical model, which is inappropriate for this approach. A consultative style replaces a chain of command, where the most appropriate professional for the needs of the moment is the one assuming primary responsibility. According to Weatherhead, the pastor should first seek to meet with the doctor in order to understand the patient's needs. In the model proposed here, the pastor might want to meet with the nurse as well.

The discussion so far has dealt with the informal, individual relationships between the physician and the pastor. There are also more formal approaches such as the development of a new discipline called "pastoral medicine," a term coined by Niedermeyer: "By pastoral medicine we mean the complete bordering sphere between medicine and theology: In the first place pastoral and moral theology, including their dogmatic basis, which results from the common need found in the practical work of both the spiritual adviser and the physician."[30] Pastoral medicine entails a certain method of research, but is also concerned with moral standards and values; the supernatural state is recognized as a reality.

Additionally, specific models are based on the cooperation between medicine and religion, physician and pastor, hospital and church, for example, in the 1980s the former Ombersley Road Surgery in Birmingham, England (now the Balsam-Heath Bird/Walji Practice), and the Wholistic Health Care Centers in the United States. In fact, in these models the nurse practitioner becomes the central professional. One of the problems in developing models for physician/nurse/pastor/patient cooperation is our health care system's individualistic and bureaucratic orientation. The only available approaches seem to depend on either an institutional structure that necessitates an interdisciplinary team of professionals, which is expensive and impractical to duplicate, or models that depend on the sensitivity and religious commitment of the physicians who would welcome contact with a pastor. (Such doctors may be rare.)

Part of the difficulty in recommending referral and cooperation between pastor, nurse, and physician on the practical level is their lack of experience in a three-way working relationship. Attempts to do this may result in great disappointment on one side or another. In a conversation held with David Cook, chaplain of Green College of Oxford University in 1991, he pointed out that the medical students he teaches may be very enthusiastic about consulting with their local vicars about patients, only to meet with unresponsiveness or the inability to respond on the part of the pastors. After several futile tries, the medical student often desists from such overtures to the church.

How can these situations be avoided? In the greater scheme of things, we need a different approach to theological, nursing, and medical education. A pattern such as that of the Ombersley Road Surgery in the 1970s and 1980s, which placed theology students in a general medical practice and medical students as interns in local churches, can go a long way toward building understanding and experience between medicine and religion. Sensitized and broadened in their view of each other's disciplines, the students could impact their respective professions.

In the 1980s I taught courses on the church's role in health care. These were cross-listed at the medical, nursing, pharmacy, and divinity schools at Howard University, and provided an interesting pilot for interdisciplinary learning; the students learned as much from one another as they did from the professor. The number of students who would select such an experience would be small, but could become leaven in the loaf. Scholarship incentives would help to launch this initially, and publicity would be crucial to enlist student participation. The Carter Center health/religion initiatives at five academic centers in the United States in the late 1990s may provide yet another model. Clinical pastoral education programs, hospital pastoral care departments, hospices, and even patient advocacy committees have fostered understanding among professionals. The newly emerging parish nurse training and degree programs are also providing models for introducing theology into the education of health care professionals.

In addition to these long-range approaches, seminars and conferences that involve practicing clergy and physicians can break down barriers of mistrust and hesitancy. Severe misunderstanding sometimes operates on both sides. Clergy are thought to be interested only in faith healing or their own church members. Physicians are assumed to worship science and reject God and personal faith as irrelevant.

Perhaps the most fruitful line of developing cooperation between physician/pastor/nurse/patient is working together within the context of a supportive and compassionate community. This relationship is important not only for patients with emotional or spiritual problems, but also for those with physical ailments. These persons may be unable to care for bodily needs or the daily chores of living, as well as experiencing the psychologically debilitating side effects of illness. For professionals, the community is an important extension of their individual support for one another.

In a transient and rootless culture, where daily contact with lifelong friends is rare and cohesive neighborhoods are swallowed up in urban planning and ribbons of freeways connecting cities and suburbs, this need for a supportive community is vital. The best type of community may be a religious one. It brings together people of varying ages and often of diverse cultural and social backgrounds, but contains an ongoing cohesiveness due to a shared set of beliefs. This does not mean that secular communities cannot fulfill some of these needs, and they do, as city social service agencies reflect, but they may not do so as effectively. The cooperation between the pastor and the parish nurse, as a new model, reflects cooperation at its best.

Pastor and Parish Nurse Collaboration

A parish nurse is a registered or licensed nurse who generally works on the staff of a local church or hospital relating to a congregation. It is one of the fastest-growing nursing specialties and now provides a model for pastor-nurse collaboration. It is crucial for a parish nurse to be part of the church staff in order to give her credibility with the congregation: committees may come and go, but a staff member is regarded more seriously. A parish nurse knows she has arrived when her name is listed under the names of the pastor and the deacons in the church bulletin and on the church letterhead. Some parish nurses meet with the pastor on a weekly basis, especially to discuss whom they have visited, and attend staff meetings and retreats. Together they decide on course of action, working as a team to try to bring a person to a healthier place in life spiritually and physically. As a team, the pastor and the parish nurse can ride on each other's coattails: if the parish nurse sees a patient she thinks is in need of deeper spiritual direction than she is equipped to provide, she alerts the pastor; if after a home visit the pastor is concerned that a person is not receiving proper care, or has a physical ailment, the pastor can call the situation to the attention of the parish nurse.

This need for a collaborative style was precisely the motivating factor to start a parish nursing program at one church in Pennsylvania where the pastor was making regular visits to a homebound church member only to discover that she was missing the cues of the church member's failing eyesight, which signaled advanced diabetes. The church member had to have her legs amputated because of her untreated diabetes, a situation that could have been prevented had a parish nurse been on staff to recognize the red flags. However, it is not always the parish nurse who saves the day.

The pastor can offer the parish nurse perspective on what it means to heal, curbing the nurse's desire to cure and helping her negotiate thorny theodicy questions. When the physician can do no more to heal the ill person, the task of caring for the patient is not over. As patients struggle to adapt to their limitations and pain, the parish nurse and the pastor are there to assist in that adaptation. In the face of suffering, all healers need one another's support. The doctor who pronounces the illness to be incurable, the patient who must adjust to the news, the parish nurse who cares, and the pastor who prays for healing are equally in need of God's grace. The key element that separates the parish nurse from other public health or community health educators may be her freedom within the religious community to emphasize and enhance the spiritual dimensions of health. At this point the cooperation between the parish nurse and the pastor is most fruitful.

Conclusion: Called to Be Agents of Healing

This book has argued that a radical reform of health care needs to embrace a more wholistic vision of health, healing, and healers. Judeo-Christian theology provides this broader vision by the understanding of health as wholeness, healing as embracing all means, activities, and forms that move us toward wholeness, and healers as coadventurers for health.

However, it is not only theology as a discipline, but the application of its wholistic vision in individual Christian lives and in the church that will ultimately transform the health care system. My companion volume discusses in detail the role of the church as a health care institution and a healing community. This book will conclude with a call to all Christians to be healing agents that bears witness to the truth that health care is more than medicine and money.

In a very special way individual Christians are called to a healing ministry. Christians are not the source but the agents of healing. As knowledge enables physicians to be special channels of God's healing power, so faith in God enables Christians to be a means of healing. The Christian may share on an intellectual level a clear value system, a raison d'être, and a doctrine of human nature that provides an integrated worldview. This may contribute to health in addition to serving the patient's concrete needs. The call to be an agent of God's healing power is central to what it means to be a Christian. Spiritual resources sustain those in suffering, give hope to those in despair, and add meaning to life for those in depression. As we show compassion and openness to the pain of others and share the transcendent in the face of the transient, we fulfill Christ's command to heal.

The Christian's contribution to health care should be marked by concern for the person in need, regardless of age, sex, race, ethnicity, physical ability, sexual orientation, or socioeconomic status. The health and healing ministry of the church is a way of glorifying God through meeting people's needs; this ministry may ultimately stand or fall on our ability to reach out in compassion to those who are suffering. No person is a healer but simply a person who cooperates with God. Christians should not refer to spiritual and physical healing. There is really only one healing.

Seven characteristics describe the individual Christian's ministry of healing: (1) consecrated, (2) courageous, (3) comprehensive, (4) communal, (5) covenantal, (6) compassionate, and (7) charitable.

The first characteristic of a healer is to be consecrated. To consecrate is to make sacred, to dedicate or to set oneself apart to God. A person first dedicates himself to service to God and then is consecrated in a worship service by the religious community. (However, this final liturgical act is not a necessity.) A consecrated individual is committed first to God, then to other persons. Consecration then has a spiritual dimension as well as a sacrificial one. These concepts are intertwined in the meaning of "consecrated." People are consecrated as peacemakers, bearers of *shalom*. In the Christian Scriptures, the concept of *eirēnē* (peace) involves making whole, bringing together persons who are alienated or angry, which is as important a dimension of healing as physical cure or care.

Being spiritual means being consecrated to God, relying on and witnessing to God as the source of all healing in our lives. This does not necessarily mean praying for special gifts of healing or charisma, but becoming an instrument of God's healing. We need both to empty ourselves so that God can work through us and to accept ourselves, or be at home with who we are so that God can open us to others and their needs.[1] The marks of consecration are humility and the offering of oneself to God, who energizes one for service, not a reliance on one's gifts and skills. We witness to God, the source of all healing.

Another aspect of consecration involves being sacrificial—becoming broken so that others may become whole. This type of sacrifice may involve visiting someone whose child has just died, which may remind us of the recent death of our own son, giving up our free time, or even risking our own health through long hours of caring for those with contagious diseases or a seriously ill family member.

Being sacrificial is what Bonhoeffer describes as costly grace,[2] not garnering accolades but bearing exhaustion for the sake of others. Apparent failure and vulnerability may be the only rewards. Our ability to sustain this discipleship comes from the refreshment of God's Spirit, which is why the sacrificial and spiritual sides of the healer are so closely connected.

The model for sacrificial healing is Christ himself, who suffered to heal— the Wounded Healer. He suffered in his temptations not to display his miraculous powers, overwhelm, or rule. He suffered in his loneliness: "Foxes have holes, and birds of the air have nests, but the Son of Man has nowhere to lay his head" (Matt. 8:20). "Christ the Healer did not only suffer as he healed; he suffered in order to heal."[3]

The second characteristic of a healer is courage. Aquinas defined courage as grace under pressure. For Aristotle it was the golden mean between foolhardiness and fear. You may stand to fight the lion, but you do not put your head in its mouth. Being courageous means taking risks, having a vision, and most of all trusting that ultimately God is in charge.

Jonathan Sacks, chief rabbi of the United Hebrew Congregation of the Commonwealth, captures this meaning of courage in recounting the historic meeting on September 13, 1995, when Yitzhak Rabin and Yasir Arafat shook hands on the White House lawn in a momentous gesture of peace. He describes the violently mixed reactions to an Israeli prime minister shaking hands with the leader of the Palestinian Liberation Organization, which had been responsible for brutal terrorist attacks. Some Jews questioned whether it was an act of statesmanship or simply of betrayal. Sacks reminds us of the story of Jacob and Esau (Gen. 32–33). Jacob prepared to meet Esau, who had earlier sworn to kill him, but then they met and kissed each other. Sacks looks not at the political or military implications but at the spiritual ones; he concludes that in Judaism, peace is a supreme value and one must sometimes take risks to secure it. Little did Sacks realize that courageous risk taking would cost Rabin his life. Jewish history is one of struggling for peace.

The mandate for peace then stems from the roots of Judaism and is part of Jewish law. "When you draw near to a town to fight against it, offer it terms of peace" (Deut. 20:10). Sacks points out that in Hebrew there are two words for "strength," *koach* and *gevurah*. *Koach* means strength to overcome your enemies. *Gevurah* means strength to overcome yourself, as in self-restraint. *Koach* is strength to wage war. *Gevurah* is strength to make peace.[4]

The third characteristic of a healer is to be comprehensive or wholistic in the way one relates to others. Like the good Samaritan, one ministers to the full needs of the person. If the healing ministry belongs to the church as well as to all individual Christians, all resources should be available for people's needs: prayer, medicine, surgery, humor, rest, exercise, diet, the sacraments, visitation. All means may be equally used by God to bring health and healing into people's lives. However, being wholistic in our ministry to others does not necessarily mean that we do everything ourselves. Obviously, each person does not have all the expertise; one needs to find those who can assist with the spiritual, emotional, physical, and mental needs of others as one reaches out in a healing ministry.

The fourth characteristic of a healer is being communal. We acknowledge that we are part of a larger community beyond the bounds of city, country, and church but also part of Christ's church universal, both visible and invisible. When we are communal, we acknowledge the support and sustenance received from others. We are connected, interrelated, and part of a *koinonia*.

Healing involves moving people from isolation, loneliness, and alienation into a supportive community.

The fifth mark of a healer is one who is covenantal; this involves a bonding with the person in need—a commitment to be with the person in all circumstances without limits. There is no contract for services but a covenant with a person to be present, both in anticipated and in unexpected situations. One should note the important distinction that W. F. May makes between code, contract, and covenant in this regard. This covenantal model, however, carries the risk of hubris and burnout. It is important to have times apart from the sick or needy; times with the vigorous and healthy; and times alone. Jesus went away from the multitudes for spiritual renewal and physical rest to reenergize the core of his being. Although being covenantal inherently means being without limits, given our human frailties, we must acknowledge the need for some boundaries to prevent burnout and disenchantment. This highlights the tension between personal needs and community concerns. Yet in crises, we may need to lay aside our own best interest for the sake of others.

The sixth characteristic of a healer is being compassionate. An aspect of compassion is a desire for justice for the poor through sharing resources for their needs. This desire stems from our understanding of equality. Since all persons have dignity and worth as children of God, no one should be denied the basic needs of life. Justice means changing the underlying structures of society that prevent all people from receiving the basics of food, shelter, health care, and clothing.

We need to confront exploitation, injustice, and prejudice, and we need to stand with those in need. Advocacy and action are elements of theology as praxis, which is rooted in our context. As one is moved by compassion, one becomes an advocate for the poor. Gustavo Gutiérrez stated that this advocacy stems from God's preferential option for the poor.[5]

Another aspect of compassion is the ability to suffer with one's neighbor. The healer must be sympathetic and also suffer to bring healing to others. This is not a passive acceptance but standing with those who are suffering. Suffering is part of the lot of being human. Compassion entails experiencing something of the predicament of illness, its anxieties, its temptations, and its assault on the whole person. Illness produces vulnerability and alienation from healthy persons. Pellegrino expresses it this way: "Every sick person is my brother or sister."[6] For the Christian, compassion is different since it stems from obedience to God, not just from unselfish motives. Compassion is probably best measured in terms of listening and acting and rarely in speaking. Even Christ asked the disciples to watch and pray with him in the Garden of Gethsemane before his crucifixion.

The fruit of compassion is the easing of loneliness, not the removing of pain. Someone who is dying from a terminal illness, grieving over the death of an only child, or having feelings of depression over the loss of a job experiences isolation and brokenness. The wound at first is gaping and intensely painful. Time brings healing as one moves from isolation to community, but the dull ache remains, ready to flare up at the most unexpected provocations.

Compassion received from another gives us hope, the hope that pain is not the end of life and that there is at least one person waiting for us. Thousands of people commit suicide because nobody is waiting for them tomorrow. We see this reflected in two of the largest groups at risk for suicide, young adults and elderly persons—young adults because of low self-esteem and pressure to excel and elderly persons because of loneliness, illness, and a sense of uselessness. There is no reason to live if there is nobody to live for. An added blessing of compassion is that as we reach out to heal others, we ourselves are healed. "We are greatest as we stoop to serve; we are tallest when we kneel to pray."[7]

Compassion requires a centering on the other, a withdrawing of self that creates space for the other to enter. To do this, one's life needs to be anchored in God. One needs to be attuned to the stirring of oneself so one can put one's needs in proper perspective. One can call this "being at home" in one's own house. Placing one's needs, worries, and tensions into proper perspective sometimes may mean taking care of oneself. This flip side of hospitality often is missing, causing anger, burnout, and even hatred. If one fails to acknowledge one's needs, deep resentments may fester inside one. Loving one's neighbor as oneself means precisely that, caring for oneself.

Compassion brings healing by creating a community of concern that communicates one is not alone in pain, someone understands, someone cares, someone is present to help. The compassionate person brings with her a total acceptance. She relaxes us. In her presence we begin to feel a change, to feel more real, more whole. She loves us with our weakness, our disabilities, our needs. The compassionate person opens her heart to others. A shared pain is no longer paralyzing.

A caring family can transform lives and the world in which we live. Transformation of lives is the fruit of compassion. Reference has been made to both prevention and intervention as two aspects of compassion. Where compassion exists, for example, the return of the elderly person to the adult child's home may lessen the negative effects of this intergenerational living.

The last mark of the healer is charitableness. Charity in the King James translation of the Bible is used to translate *agape,* the unselfish, complete love of God. This love is described in 1 Corinthians 13 as patient, kind, not boastful or envious, free from pride, and not self-seeking. This view of love is seen through Christ's life: "This is my commandment, that you love one another as I have loved you. No one has greater love than this, to lay down one's life for one's friends. You are my friends if you do what I command you" (John 15:12–14). My hope is that this book is a call for this self-giving love at the heart of true health care reform; that we may experience healing in our own lives as well as be agents of healing for others.

NOTES

INTRODUCTION

1. "Wholistic" refers to integrated health care that draws on spiritual and scientific resources in the mainstream of medicine and religion. It is distinguished from "holistic" health care, which generally eschews traditional medicine and follows more controversial health care practices.

2. U.S. Bureau of the Census, *Statistical Abstract of the United States, 1996,* 116th ed. (Washington, D.C., 1996), 120. In 1994, there were about 40 million people in the United States not covered by health insurance, representing about 15 percent of the population. The profile of the uninsured American shows a distinction by sex of 21.3 million men and 18.4 million women; by race, 30.3 million white, 6.6 million black, and the balance Hispanic and other races; by age, 10 million under the age of eighteen years, 9.1 million between twenty-five and thirty-four years, 6.8 million between thirty-five and forty-four years, 6.7 million between eighteen and twenty-four years, 3.9 million between forty-five and fifty-four years, 2.9 million between fifty-five and sixty-four years, and 300,000, sixty-five years and older. Regionally, the ten states with the highest percentage of residents not covered by health insurance were Texas, New Mexico, California, Arizona, Alabama, Louisiana, Mississippi, Oklahoma, Arkansas, and Florida.

HEALTH CARE IN CRISIS

1. U.S. Senate Labor and Human Resources Committee and Senate Finance Committee, "The Health Insurance Portability and Accountability Act," Summary, File H.R. 3103, photocopy.

2. "Editorial," *Times* (London), 21 April 1996, CC3.

3. Madison Powers, "Justice and the Market for Health Issues: Current Proposals for Securing Access to Health Care" (paper presented at the Kennedy Institute of Ethics, Washington, D.C., 21 March 1991).

4. "AMA/Gallup Survey Reveals Public's Attitudes on Health System Reform," *Michigan Medicine* 93, no. 6 (June 1994): 15–19.

5. Ibid., 16.

6. Martina Darragh and Pat Milmoe McCarrick, "Managed Health Care: New Ethical Issues for All," *Kennedy Institute of Ethics Journal* 6, no. 2, Scope Note 31, Baltimore: Johns Hopkins University Press (June 1996): 189–92.

7. Larry Lipman, "The Medicare Battle Rages On," *Trenton Times,* 4 April 1997, A13.

8. Ibid., 2.

9. Charles Andrews, *Profit Fever: The Drive of Corporatized Health Care and How to Stop It* (Monroe, Maine: Common Courage Press, 1995), 5.

10. Ibid., 7.

11. Ibid., 11.

12. Robert Kuttner, "Mutant HMOs," *Washington Post*, 1 January 1997, A19.

13. Ibid.

14. Susan Dentzer, "Shedding Light on Managed Care," *U.S. News and World Report*, 6 May 1996, 120.

15. "Health Care Spending Projected to Double in Decade," September 14, 1998 (Washington, D.C.: Associated Press, 1998), CNN Interactive (http://cnn.com/HEALTH/9809/14/health.care.spending.ap) (September 22, 1998).

16. George Anders, "The Outlook for HMOs," April 14, 1998, Frontline Online (http://www.pbs.org/wgbh/pages/frontline/shows/hmo/etc/outlook.html) (September 22, 1998).

17. Dentzer, "Shedding Light on Managed Care," 120.

18. George Anders, "A Profile of Malik Hasan," April 14, 1998, Frontline Online (http://www.pbs.org/wgbh/pages/frontline/shows/hmo/hassan/profile.html) (September 22, 1998).

19. InterStudy Publications, Publications and Services Catalog (Saint Paul: Decision Resources) (winter 1996): 3–7.

20. Ronald J. Glasser, M.D., "The Doctor Is Not In," *Harper's Magazine*, March 1998, 39.

21. Stuart Auerbach, "Managed Care Backlash," *Washington Post*, Health Section, 25 June 1996, 12–15.

22. Glasser, "The Doctor Is Not In," 40.

23. Nationally, out-of-pocket health expenditures totaled $174.9 billion in 1994. See Bureau of the Census, *Statistical Abstract of the United States*, 1996, 112.

24. Auerbach, "Managed Care Backlash," 14.

25. "Poll: American Anxious about Health Care System," February 28, 1998 (Washington, D.C.: CNN, 1998), CNN Interactive (http://cnn.com/HEALTH/9802/28/health.poll) (September 22, 1998).

26. Glasser, "The Doctor Is Not In," 37.

27. Kuttner, "Mutant HMOs," A19.

28. Ibid., 35.

29. InterStudy Publications, Publications and Services Catalog, 5.

30. Amitai Etzioni, "One Fuming Physician," *Washington Post*, 17 September 1995, C3.

31. "A Bill of Health," February 5, 1998, Online News Hour (http://www.pbs.org/newshour/bb/health) (September 30, 1998).

32. Glasser, "The Doctor Is Not In," 78.

33. Edmund Pellegrino, "Managed Care and Managed Competition: Some Ethical Reflections," *Calyx* 4, no. 4 (1994): 1–5.

34. Auerbach, "Managed Care Backlash," 15.

35. Erik Larson, "The Soul of an HMO," *Time*, 22 January 1996, 45.

36. Edmund Pellegrino, "Words Can Hurt You: Some Reflections on the Metaphors of Managed Care" (First Annual Nicholas J. Pisacano Lecture), *Journal of the American Board of Family Practice* (November–December 1994): 505.

37. John H. Fielder, "Disposable Doctors: Incentives to Abuse Physician Peer Review," *Journal of Clinical Ethics* 6, no. 4 (winter 1995): 331.

38. Auerbach, "Managed Care Backlash," 14.

39. "Health Care Spending Projected to Double in Decade" [September 22, 1998].

40. Judi Hasson, "Doctors' Incomes Up 6.7 Percent after '94 Drop"; Hasson and Steven Findlay, "Signs Hint at Higher Health Costs," *USA Today*, 20 December 1996, 1, 3A.

41. "Health Care Spending Projected to Double in Decade" [September 22, 1998].

42. Steven A. Schroeder, "Cost Containment in U.S. Health Care," summary in Darragh and McCarrick, "Managed Health Care," 189–92.

43. Laurie Zoloth-Dorfman and Susan Rubin, "The Patient as Commodity: Managed Care and the Question of Ethics," *Journal of Clinical Ethics* 6, no. 4 (winter 1995): 347.

44. Andrews, *Profit Fever*, 24.

45. Don Colburn, "Nurses' Jobs Are Changing or Disappearing," *Washington Post Health*, 22 November 1994, 8.

46. Andrews, *Profit Fever*, 24.

47. Darragh and McCarrick, "Managed Health Care," 191.

48. David Azevedo, "Rationing: America—From De Facto to Explicit," *Medical Economics*, 24 May 1993, 184–90, 196–99.

49. David Azevedo, "Are We Asking Too Much of Gatekeepers?" *Medical Economics*, 11 April 1994, 126, 128, 130–32, 134–37.

50. Ibid., 128.

51. Azevedo, "Rationing," 187.

52. "How Good Is Your Health Plan?" *Consumer Reports*, August 1996, 36.

53. Sharon J. Jackson, "Why Managed Care, Why Now?" *Journal of the California Alliance for the Mentally Ill* 7, no. 1 (1 April 1996): 6.

54. Associated Press, "Coverage of Preventive Care Endorsed by Health Insurer," *Washington Post*, 19 June 1991, A3.

2. The Focus on Medical Care

1. Miriam Siegler and Humphry Osmond, *Models of Madness, Models of Medicine* (New York: Macmillan, 1974), 23.

2. George Engel, "The Need for a New Medical Model: A Challenge for Biomedicine," in *Concepts of Health and Disease: Interdisciplinary Perspectives*, ed. Arthur Caplan, H. Tristram Engelhardt Jr., and James McCartney (Reading, Mass.: Addison-Wesley, 1981), 591.

3. Gary Albrecht, "Social Aspects of Medical Care: Conceptual Approaches to the Field," in *Health, Illness, and Medicine*, ed. Gary Albrecht and Paul Higgins (Chicago: Rand McNally, 1979), 10.

4. Stephen Pattison, *Alive and Kicking* (London: SCM Press, 1993), 22. A popular alternative to this model is the psychological perspective on illness. There are many illustrations of psychosomatic illness. Emotions, for example, have physiological reactions of an angry person turning red, a frightened person turning white, anxiety inflaming the lining of the stomach. Also recent studies show how character type may affect an illness. Bereaved people are more vulnerable to disease and death. So new attitudes and practices are recommended. The remedies suggested tend to be with individuals to help them relax. However, this can lead to blaming a person for her illness, something that more socially oriented analyses of disease try to avoid.

5. Robert Veatch, "The Medical Model: Its Nature and Problems," in *Concepts of Health and Disease*, 544.

6. Ibid., 530.

7. Eliot Friedson, *Profession of Medicine* (New York: Dodd, Mead, 1975), 233.

8. Veatch, "The Medical Model," 524.

9. Engel, "The Need for a New Medical Model," 591.

10. Ibid., 594, 598. Engel's biopsychosocial model appears to blur the distinction between illness and problems of living and places too heavy a burden on the physician. In his self-described patient- rather than illness-centered treatment, the physician must evaluate the patient's overall problems and refer her to the appropriate professionals.

11. See Horacio Fabrega, "Concepts of Disease: Logical Features and Social Implications," in *Concepts of Health and Disease,* 493–522.

12. Siegler and Osmond, *Models of Medicine,* 90. This book discusses T. T. Paterson's view.

13. See chapter 3 for a discussion of Asclepius and Asclepian authority.

14. Mark Siegler, "The Doctor-Patient Encounter and Its Relationship to Theories of Health and Disease," in *Concepts of Health and Disease,* 634.

15. Talcott Parsons, *The Social System* (New York: Free Press, 1951), 428–79.

16. Siegler and Osmond, *Models of Medicine,* 99.

17. Ibid., 24.

18. Veatch, "The Medical Model," 541.

19. Ibid., 523.

20. Ibid.

21. Siegler and Osmond, *Models of Medicine,* 89.

22. Renée Fox, "The Medicalization and Demedicalization of American Society," in *Doing Better and Feeling Worse,* ed. John Knowles (New York: Norton, 1977), 10.

23. Quoted in ibid., 11.

24. U.S. Bureau of the Census, *Historical Statistics of the United States, Colonial Times to 1970,* bicentennial ed., pt. 2, 56.

25. U.S. Bureau of the Census, *Statistical Abstract of the United States,* 1995, 115th ed. (Washington, D.C., 1995), 90.

26. United Kingdom in Figures 1996 Edition (http://www.ons.gov.uk/ukinfigs/stats/pop.html).

3. PROBLEMS IN THE MEDICAL MODEL

1. Leon Kass, "Regarding the End of Medicine and the Pursuit of Health," in *Concepts of Health and Disease,* 13.

2. Pattison, *Alive and Kicking,* 29.

3. Ibid., 42.

4. James C. McGilvray, ed., *The Quest for Health and Wholeness* (Tübingen: German Institute for Medical Missions, 1981), 82.

5. Ibid., 83.

6. Pattison, *Alive and Kicking,* 26.

7. Ray Capone, "Conceptual Problems in Defining Health" (paper presented at Kennedy Institute of Ethics Seminar, n.d.), 6.

8. McGilvray, *The Quest for Health,* 86. This definition was updated in mid-1998 and spiritual well-being was added.

9. Daniel Callahan, in *Doing Better and Feeling Worse,* 26.

10. Elsie L. Bandman and Bertram Bandman, "Health and Disease: A Nursing Perspective," in *Concepts of Health and Disease,* 686.

11. Leon Kass, "The Hippocratic Oath: Thoughts on Medicine and Ethics" (lecture presented at University of Chicago, 12 November 1980), 29.

12. McGilvray, *The Quest for Health,* 82.

13. René Dubos, *The Mirage of Health* (New York: Harper & Row, 1979), 129–30.

14. Ibid.

15. Ibid., 130.

16. Ibid., 135.

17. The median annual salary for doctors is $156,000 and for nurses $40,900. Timothy Begany, "1995 Earnings Survey: The News Is Mixed," *RN* 58, no. 10 (October 1995): 49.

18. Veatch, "The Medical Model," 533.

19. Gerald May, *Addiction and Grace* (San Francisco: Harper & Row, 1988).

20. See Thomas Szasz, "The Myth of Mental Illness," *American Psychologist* 15 (February 1960): 113–18.

21. Veatch, "The Medical Model," 539.

22. Paul Wymer, "They Also Learn Who Only Sit and Wait," *Times Educational Supplement,* 6 September 1996, 25.

23. Fox, "The Medicalization and Demedicalization," 13.

24. Health Reference Center abstract from *American Medical News,* 15 April 1996, 11.

25. William F. May, "Code, Covenant, and Contract," *Hastings Center Report* 35 (December 1975): 32.

26. Mark Siegler (lecture presented at Royal Society of London, Conference on Managed Care, Washington, D.C., June 1997).

27. Lewis Thomas (address presented at Rose F. Kennedy Lecture Series, Georgetown University, Washington, D.C., January 1983).

28. Fox, "The Medicalization and Demedicalization," 17–18.

29. Ibid., 19.

30. Ibid.

31. Michael Wilson, *Health Is for People* (London: Darton, Longman & Todd, 1975), 13.

32. National Center for Health Statistics, *National Hospital Discharge Survey, Annual Summary* (Washington, D.C.: U.S. Government Printing Office, 1993), 14.

33. Veatch, "The Medical Model," 530.

34. Andrews, *Profit Fever,* 23.

35. "Chronic Care in America: A 21st Century Challenge," prepared by the Institute for Health and Aging, University of California, San Francisco, for the Robert Wood Johnson Foundation, Princeton, New Jersey, 1996, 9. "Chronic conditions is a general term that includes chronic illnesses and impairments. Chronic illness is the presence of long-term disease or symptoms."

36. Ibid., 14–15. "Given the limits of medical and public health knowledge at the beginning of this century, Americans frequently died at young ages from infectious and parasitic diseases. As sanitation, nutrition, and living conditions improved and medical technology advanced, deaths from infectious diseases declined steadily and children and young adults survived longer. While deaths from infectious diseases have decreased, deaths from chronic conditions have increased. The changes statistically are: in 1900 infectious diseases accounted for 30 percent of deaths and in 1990 5.3 percent; in 1900 cardiovascular disease accounted for 20.1 percent of deaths and in 1990 42 percent."

37. Ibid., 17.

38. Ibid., 42.

39. Ibid., 52.

40. G. W. Strahan, "An Overview of Nursing Homes and Their Current Residents: Data from the 1995 National Nursing Home Survey," Advance Data from Vital and Health Statistics no. 280 (Hyattsville, Md.: National Center for Health Statistics, 1970), 2–3.

41. "Closing the Gap," in *Striving for Fullness of Life: The Church's Challenge in Health* (Atlanta: Carter Center of Emory University Conference, 25–27 October 1989), 8. The percentages given here exceed 100 percent as reported.

42. Bureau of the Census, *Statistical Abstract of the United States, 1996,* 96.

43. "Closing the Gap," 7.

44. Michael McGinnis and William Foege, "Actual Causes of Death in the United States," *Journal of the American Medical Association* 270 (10 November 1993): 2207.

45. The White House Office of National Drug Control Policy (Washington, D.C.: U.S. Government Printing Office, June 1997).

46. McGilvray, *The Quest for Health,* 15.

47. Dubos, *The Mirage of Health*, 24.

48. Rick Carlson quoted in Fox, "The Medicalization and Demedicalization," 20.

49. Paul Ramsey, conversation with author, 1974.

50. William Middleton, *Values in Modern Medicine* (Madison: Wisconsin University Press, 1972), 227.

51. See Richard Katz, *The Boiling Energy* (Cambridge: Harvard University Press, 1982), for a study of this phenomenon among the Kalahari Kung.

52. Ivan Illich, *Medical Nemesis* (London: Calder and Boyars, 1975), 165.

53. Ivan Illich, *Medical Nemesis* (New York: Pantheon Books, 1976), 3. "Iatrogenesis" is "the disabling impact of professional control over medicine."

54. Ibid., 121.

55. Veatch, "The Medical Model," 537.

56. Ibid., 15.

57. McGilvray, *The Quest for Health*, 14.

58. Wilson, *Health Is for People*, 27.

59. Ivan Illich, "Brave New Biocracy: A Critique of Health Care from Womb to Tomb," in *Ecology of Health: Identifying Issues and Alternatives*, ed. Jennifer Chesworth (Thousand Oaks, Calif.: Sage Publications, 1996), 18.

60. Illich, *Medical Nemesis* (London: Calder & Boyars, 1975), xiii. See also *Deschooling Society* (New York: Harper & Row, 1971).

61. Ibid. (London edition), xiv.

62. Illich, *Ecology of Health*, 18.

63. Ibid., 26.

64. Ibid., 121.

65. Ibid., 73–84.

66. Ibid., 74–75.

67. Illich quoted in Fox, "The Medicalization and Demedicalization," 10.

68. Illich, *Ecology of Health*, 24.

69. See William A. Nolen, *Healing: A Doctor in Search of a Miracle* (New York: Random House, 1974), for an exposé of the Philippine psychic surgeons.

70. Williard Gaylin, "Faulty Diagnosis," *New York Times*, 12 June 1994, 4A, 1.

71. Fay J. Ellis, "Academics Explore Spirituality and Medicine," *Academic Physician and Scientist* (March/April 1998): 8. Published by Association of American Medical Colleges.

72. "Advance: Top Medical Schools Receive Awards to Teach Spirituality and Health," NewsPage information service (Individual Inc.) from *Business Wire*, 27 August 1996.

73. R. L. Dickman, R. E. Sarnacki, F. T. Schimpfhauser, and L. A. Katz, "Medical Students from Natural Science and Non-Science Undergraduate Backgrounds," *Journal of the American Medical Association* 243 (27 June 1980): 2506.

74. S. G. Wolf, "I Can't Afford a B," *New England Journal of Medicine* 299 (1978): 949–50.

75. Harrison G. Gough, "The Recruitment and Selection of Medical Students," in *Psychosocial Aspects of Medical Training*, ed. R. H. Coombs and C. H. Vincent (Springfield: Charles C. Thomas Publisher, 1971); J. M. Rhoads, H. L. Gallemore, D. T. Gianturco, et al., "Motivation, Medical School Admissions and Student Performance," *Journal of Medical Education* 49 (1974): 1119–27.

76. Abraham Flexner, *Medical Education in the U.S. and Canada* (New York: Arno Press, 1972), 25–26.

77. Dickman et al., "Medical Students," 2506–9.

78. Steven Jonas, *Medical Mystery: The Training of Doctors in the U.S.* (New York: Norton, 1978), 274, and Marcel Fredericks and Paul Mundy, *The Making of a Physician: A Ten Year Longitudinal Study of Social Class, Academic Achievement, and Changing Professional Attitudes of a Medical School Class* (Chicago: Loyola University Press, 1976).

79. Abigail Rian Evans, "Does the Undergraduate Study of Humanities Jeopardize Medical Students?" (study, Admissions Office of College of Physicians and Surgeons, Columbia University, New York, New York, 1981).

80. Abigail Rian Evans, "Admissions Criteria for Medical School Which Consider Ethical Sensitivity and Service Orientation" (study, College of Physicians and Surgeons, Columbia University, New York, New York, August 1982). This study developed a list of eleven moral attributes and reviewed applicants' interviews and letters of reference to see if they were mentioned.

81. Some medical schools were seeking to make such changes as evidenced by a study done at the College of Physicians and Surgeons at Columbia University, New York, New York, 1979–81, by Abigail Evans to develop criteria for admissions to medical school that would take into account ethical sensitivity and service orientation in medical school applicants.

82. Malcolm Rigler, interview with author, Withymoor Village Surgery, Birmingham, England, 28 October 1996. According to Dr. Rigler, the urgency of the need for arts and health initiatives has been advocated most persuasively by Dr. Petr Skrabanek in *The Death of Humane Medicine and the Rise of Coercive Healthism.*

83. Wymer, "They Also Learn Who Only Sit and Wait," 25.

84. Bureau of the Census, *Statistical Abstract of the United States,* 1996, 111–12. This is the source for all the following data on health care spending.

85. Paul G. Ginsburg and Jon R. Gabel, "Tracking Health Care Costs: What's New in 1998?" *Health Affairs* 17, no. 5 (September/October 1998): 142.

86. "Chronic Care in America: A 21st Century Challenge," 9.

87. Health Care Task Force, Briefing (Washington, D.C.: U.S. Government Printing Office, 1993), 45.

88. Ibid.

89. U.S. Bureau of the Census, Current Population Survey (http://www.census. gov/hhcs/ www/hlthins.html) (March 1996).

90. Ibid.

91. Marshall Raffel and Norma Raffel, *The U.S. Health System: Origins and Functions,* 3d ed. (Media, Pa.: Harwal Publishing, 1989), 223.

92. Sheila Smith, Mark Freeland, Stephen Heffler, et al., "The Next Ten Years of Health Spending: What Does the Future Hold?" *Health Affairs* 17, no. 5 (September/October 1998): 128–31.

93. Ginsburg and Gabel, "Tracking Health Care Costs," 142.

94. McGinnis and Foege, "Actual Causes of Death in the United States," 2207.

95. "How Good Is Your Health Plan?" 28.

96. U.S. Bureau of the Census, Census of Population and Housing (Washington, D.C., 1990).

97. Dr. Jeremy Rogers, United Kingdom National Health Service (http://www.cs.man.ac. uk/mig/people/jeremy/nhs.html) (21 January 1998), 2.

98. Ibid., 4–7.

99. Andrews, *Profit Fever,* 44.

100. Ibid. This poll did not indicate whether it included people in health plans or not.

4. HEALTH AS MORE THAN MEDICINE AND MONEY

1. Edmund Pellegrino, "The Healing Relationship: The Architectonics of Clinical Medicine" (lecture presented at the University of Texas Health Science Center, Houston, Texas, April 1982), 22.

2. Edmund D. Pellegrino and David C. Thomasma, *A Philosophical Basis of Medical Practice* (New York: Oxford University Press, 1981), 181.

3. Christopher Boorse, "On the Distinction between Disease and Illness," in *Concepts of Health and Disease,* 545.

4. Dubos, *The Mirage of Health*, 26.

5. Pellegrino and Thomasma, *A Philosophical Basis of Medical Practice*, 181.

6. Kass, "Regarding the End of Medicine," 11.

7. Ibid., 12.

8. McGilvray, *The Quest for Health*, 86.

9. Ivan Illich, "Health as One's Own Responsibility: NO, Thank You," *Journal of Consciousness Studies* 1 (summer 1994): 26.

10. Ibid., 27.

11. Michael Ruse, "Are Homosexuals Sick?" in *Concepts of Health and Disease*, 695.

12. Talcott Parsons, "Definitions of Health and Illness in the Light of American Values and Social Structure," in *Concepts of Health and Disease*, 60.

13. H. Tristram Englehardt Jr., "The Concepts of Health and Disease," in *Concepts of Health and Disease*, 31.

14. Kass, "Regarding the End of Medicine," 30.

15. Ibid., 9.

16. Ibid., 5–6.

17. Edmund D. Pellegrino and David C. Thomasma, "Toward an Axiology for Medicine: A Response to Kazem Sadegh-Zadeh," *Metamedicine* 2 (June 1981): 336.

18. Edmund D. Pellegrino and David C. Thomasma, "Philosophy of Medicine as the Source for Medical Ethics," *Metamedicine* 2 (June 1981): 8.

19. Edmund D. Pellegrino and David C. Thomasma, "Medicine as a Science of Action: A Response to Peter Hucklenbroich," *Metamedicine* 2 (June 1981): 236.

20. Pellegrino and Thomasma, "Toward an Axiology for Medicine," 338.

21. Parsons, "Definitions of Health and Illness," 60.

22. Karl Barth, *Church Dogmatics: The Doctrine of Creation*, vol. 3, pt. 4 (London: T. & T. Clark, 1961).

23. Ralph Peterson, *A Study of the Healing Church and Its Ministry: The Health Care Apostolate* (New York: Lutheran Church in America, 1982), 7.

24. Ibid.

25. Harriet Moidel, *Nursing Care of the Patient with Medical-Surgical Disorders* (New York: McGraw Hill, 1971), 51–52.

26. Boorse, "On the Distinction between Disease and Illness," 560.

27. Ibid., 551.

28. Ibid.

29. Richard Siebeck quoted in Barth, *Church Dogmatics*, 356.

30. René Dubos quoted in Peterson, *A Study of the Healing Church*, 6.

31. Bernard Martin, *Healing for You* (Richmond: John Knox Press, 1965), 141.

32. Siebeck quoted in Barth, *Church Dogmatics*, 356.

33. Kass, "Regarding the End of Medicine," 19–20.

34. "Search for a Christian," Christian Medical Commission of the World Council of Churches (Geneva, Switzerland, 1982), 17.

35. Ibid., 18.

36. Ibid., 32.

37. Ibid., 18.

38. David Hilton, conversation with author, Atlanta, Georgia, October 1997.

39. Morris Maddocks, *The Christian Healing Ministry* (London: SPCK, 1981), 7.

40. Michael Wilson, *Health Is for People* (London: Darton, Longman, & Todd, 1975).

41. Denis Duncan, *Pastoral Care and Ethical Issues* (Edinburgh: Saint Andrew Press, 1988), 58–60.

42. Martin, *Healing for You*, 141.

Reenvisioning Health and Sickness

1. McGilvray, *The Quest for Health*, 86.
2. Though some, such as Pellegrino, suggest medicine is based on a doctrine of the perfectibility of humankind.
3. Albert Niedermeyer, *Compendium of Pastoral Medicine* (New York: I. F. Wagner, 1960), 281–86.
4. Kass, "Regarding the End of Medicine," 19–20.
5. Kenneth Vaux, "In Search of a Context and Concept of Wholistic Health," in *Theological Roots of Wholistic Health Care*, ed. Granger E. Westberg (Hinsdale, Ill.: Wholistic Health Centers, 1979), 66.
6. Nancy Tubesing, *Philosophical Assumptions* (Chicago: Wholistic Health Centers, 1977), 5.
7. Vaux, "In Search of a Context and Concept," 69.
8. "The Relation of the Christian Faith to Health," report of 172nd General Assembly of the United Presbyterian Church in the U.S.A. (Philadelphia: Office of the General Assembly, 1960), 36–37.
9. Ernest Becker, *The Revolution in Psychiatry* (New York: Free Press, 1964).
10. Ibid.
11. Craig W. Ellison, "Spiritual Well-Being: Conceptualization and Measurement," *Journal of Psychology and Theology* (fall 1983): 3.
12. A lecture given by Craig W. Ellison at the National Interfaith Coalition on Aging, 1975.
13. Viktor Frankl quoted in Ellison, "Spiritual Well-Being," 5.
14. Robert Lambourne, "Daily Round of Suffering and Healing," in *The Wonder of Divine Healing*, ed. A. A. Jones (Evesham: Arthur James, 1958), 56–67.
15. Thomas Szasz, *The Myth of Mental Illness: Foundations of a Theory of Personal Conduct* (New York: Harper & Row, 1974).
16. John Patrick Dolan and William N. Adams-Smith, *Health & Society* (New York: Seabury Press, 1978).
17. Kass, "Regarding the End of Medicine," 15.
18. Michael Wilson, "The Hospital in Society: Health, Attitudes, and Values," in *World Council of Churches Christian Medical Commission Contact Special Series*, no. 2 (Geneva: WCC, June 1979), p. 71 (www.wcc-coe.org.library).
19. R. A. Lambourne, "Wholeness, Community and Worship," in *Explorations in Health and Salvation: A Selection of Papers by Bob Lambourne*, ed. Michael Wilson (Birmingham, Eng.: University of Birmingham, 1985), 20.
20. Thomas Droege, "The Religious Roots of Wholistic Health Care," in *Theological Roots of Wholistic Health Care*, 42.
21. Paul Tournier, *A Doctor's Casebook in Light of the Bible* (New York: Harper & Row, 1960), 240.
22. "The Relation of the Christian Faith to Health," 11.
23. Tournier, *A Doctor's Casebook*, 242.
24. Ronald Spivey, "Prayer and Healing," in *Religion and Medicine*, ed. John Crowlesmith (London: Epworth Press, 1962), 114.
25. McGilvray, *The Quest for Health*, 27.
26. "The Relation of the Christian Faith to Health," 25.
27. Peterson, *A Study of the Healing Church*, 7.
28. Boorse, "On the Distinction between Disease and Illness," 546.
29. Ibid., 555.
30. Engelhardt, "The Concepts of Health and Disease," 33.
31. Ibid., 32.

32. Horacio Fabrega Jr., "The Scientific Usefulness of the Idea of Illness," in *Concepts of Health and Disease*, 131.

33. Engelhardt, "The Concepts of Health and Disease," 34, 38.

34. Parsons, "Definitions of Health and Illness," 60.

35. Lester S. King, "What Is Disease," in *Concepts of Health and Disease*, 112.

36. Barth, *Church Dogmatics*, 357.

37. Droege, "The Religious Roots of Wholistic Health Care," 40.

38. Ibid., 14.

39. D. S. Allister, *Sickness and Healing in the Church* (Oxford: Latimer House, 1981), 15.

40. *Job for Modern Man: Today's English Version* (American Bible Society, 1971) is used for a clearer meaning instead of the NRSV.

41. Leuven Institute Lectures, Belgium, summer 1996.

42. Evelyn Frost, *Christian Healing* (London: Mowbray and Co., 1940), 24.

6. Healing as Moving toward Wholeness

1. Pattison, *Alive and Kicking*, 19.

2. Frost, *Christian Healing*, 172.

3. Ibid., 173.

4. Sandy Rovner, "Healthtalk: The Nurse's Touch," *Washington Post*, 2 December 1983, D5.

5. Martin, *Healing for You*, 141.

6. Morris Maddocks, *Journey to Wholeness* (London: Highway Press, 1986), 58.

7. Trevor Nash, "Wounded Healer" (lecture notes presented at Acorn Healing Trust Retreat, Borden, England, 26 October 1996).

8. Robert A. Lambourne, "Wholeness, Community, and Worship" and "The Deliverance Map of Disease and Sin," in *Explorations in Health and Salvation*, 12–27, 98–106.

9. Ibid., 17–18.

10. Ibid.

11. Morton Enslin, *Christian Beginnings*, pts. 1 and 2 (New York: Harper & Row, 1956), 123.

12. Robert A. Lambourne, "What Is Healing?" in *Explorations in Health and Salvation*, 28.

13. Droege, "The Religious Roots of Wholistic Health Care," 42.

14. Ibid., 32.

15. Donald Coggan, *Convictions* (Grand Rapids, Mich.: Eerdmans, 1975).

16. Myung-Soo Lee, *A Treatise on Healing Ministry* (Seoul, Korea: Sung Whang, 1988), 13.

17. Lambourne, "What Is Healing?" 28–33.

18. Ibid., 30.

19. William Strawson, "The Theology of Healing," in *Religion and Medicine*, ed. Crowlesmith, 91.

20. David Smith, "Suffering, Medicine, and Christian Theology," in *On Moral Medicine: Theological Perspectives in Medical Ethics*, ed. Stephen E. Lammers and Allen Verhey (Grand Rapids, Mich.: Eerdmans, 1987), 256.

21. Ibid., 259.

22. Pierre Wolf, *May I Hate God* (New York: Paulist Press, 1979).

23. Martin Marty, *A Cry of Absence: Reflections for the Winter of the Heart* (San Francisco: Harper & Row, 1983), 2–7.

24. Ibid., 12.

25. Ibid., 8.

26. Diedra Kriewald, "Tangles—Powerlessness" and "Journey toward Wholeness," in *Hallelujah Anyhow: Suffering and the Christian Community of Faith* (New York: General Board of Global Ministries, United Methodist Church, 1986), 103, 117.

27. Smith, "Suffering, Medicine, and Christian Theology," 258.

28. Marty, *A Cry of Absence,* 103.

29. See Gustaf Aulen, *The Faith of the Christian Church* (Philadelphia: Fortress Press, 1960), for an exposition of faith and God.

30. Marty, "The Season of Abandonment," chapter 7 in *A Cry of Absence.*

31. Lambourne, "Daily Round of Suffering and Healing."

32. Maddocks, *The Christian Healing Ministry,* 9.

33. Frost, *Christian Healing,* 202.

34. Strawson, "The Theology of Healing," 94.

35. Miguel de Unamuno, *Tragic Sense of Life,* trans. J. E. Crawford Flitch (New York: Dover Publications, 1954).

36. Peter Speck, *Being There: Pastoral Care in Time of Illness* (London: SPCK, 1993), 26–28.

37. Søren Kierkegaard, *The Gospel of Suffering: The Lilies of the Field* (Minneapolis: Augsburg, 1948).

38. Charles Wallis, *The Treasure Chest* (New York: Harper & Row, 1965), 137.

39. Charles W. Gusmer, *The Ministry of Healing* (Great Wakering, Eng.: Mayhew-McCrimmon, 1974), 50.

40. Marty, *A Cry of Absence,* 125ff.

7. THE RELATIONSHIP BETWEEN FAITH AND HEALING

1. Maddocks, *The Christian Healing Ministry,* 59.

2. Lambourne, "Wholeness, Community and Worship," 12–27.

3. Pattison, *Alive and Kicking,* 80.

4. Droege, "The Religious Roots of Wholistic Health Care," 13.

5. Ibid., 45–46. Henry R. Rust, "A Pastor's Perspective on Our Wholistic Health Center," in *Theological Roots of Wholistic Health Care,* 54.

6. Droege, "The Religious Roots of Wholistic Health Care," 9.

7. Frost, *Christian Healing,* 163.

8. Duncan, *Pastoral Care and Ethical Issues,* 74. Citing Christopher Cooke.

9. Strawson, "The Theology of Healing," 105.

10. Maddocks, *The Christian Healing Ministry,* 35.

11. Erastus Evans, "The Significance of the New Testament Healing Miracles for the Modern Healer," in *Religion and Medicine,* ed. Crowlesmith, 71.

12. Howard Clark Kee, *Medicine, Miracle and Magic in New Testament Times* (New York: Cambridge University Press, 1988), 10.

13. C. Gordon Scorer and Vincent Edmunds, *Some Thoughts on Faith Healing* (London: Tyndale Press, 1956), 26.

14. Ibid., 59.

15. Maddocks, *The Christian Healing Ministry,* 77.

8. THE PATIENT AS THE CENTRAL HEALER

1. Fifty-four percent of adults and 25 percent of children are overweight. "Study: Americans Fatter Than Ever and Getting Even Fatter," May 28, 1998 (Washington, D.C.: CNN, 1998), CNN Interactive (http://CNN.com/HEALTH/9805/28/obesity) (September 30, 1998).

2. W. J. Sheils, ed., *The Church and Healing: Papers Read at the Twentieth Summer Meeting and the Twenty-First Winter Meeting of the Ecclesiastical History Society* (Oxford: Basil Blackwell, 1982), 143.

3. Ibid., 264.

4. Ibid., 177.

5. John D. Stoeckle, "Reflections on Modern Doctoring" (paper presented at the Royal Society of Medicine Conference, Washington, D.C., June 1997).

6. Ronald C. Kessler et al., "Patterns and Correlates of Self-Help Group Membership in the United States," *Social Policy* (spring 1997): 27–44.

7. Eric Cassell, *The Healer's Art* (New York: Penguin Books, 1979), 168.

8. Eric Cassell, "Reactions to Physical Illness and Hospitalization," in *Psychiatry and General Medical Practice,* ed. Gene Usdin and Jerry M. Lewis (New York: McGraw-Hill, 1979), 124.

9. Cassell, *The Healer's Art,* 33.

10. Peterson, *A Study of the Healing Church,* 7.

11. Richard Selzer quoted by Edmund Pellegrino in commencement address (University of Illinois at the Medical Center, Chicago, Illinois, 6 June 1980).

12. Leon Eisenberg, "What Makes Persons 'Patients' and Patients 'Well'?" *American Journal of Medicine* (August 1980): 279.

13. Barth, *Church Dogmatics,* 358.

14. Ibid., 363, 367.

15. Peterson, *A Study of the Healing Church,* 15.

16. Ibid.

17. Norman Cousins, *Anatomy of an Illness* (New York: Norton, 1979).

18. Tubesing, *Philosophical Assumptions,* 8.

19. Parsons, "Definitions of Health and Illness," 81.

20. Karl Menninger, cited in Edgar Jackson, *The Role of Faith in the Process of Healing* (London: SCM Press, 1981), 77.

21. David Belgum, *Religion and Medicine* (Ames: Iowa State University Press, 1967), 208.

22. Jackson, *The Role of Faith,* 79.

23. Ibid., 14.

24. Ibid., 58.

25. Ibid., 141.

26. "Holistic Medicine," *New York Times,* 25 April 1978, 43.

27. Sandy Rovner, "Healthtalk: The Rhythm of Life," *Washington Post,* 12 October 1979, B5.

28. Kim Robert Clark, "The Impact of Religious Beliefs on Compliance," monograph, Loma Linda School of Public Health, California, 2.

29. Ibid.

30. Jackson, *The Role of Faith,* 23. See A. R. Evans, forthcoming companion volume to *Redeeming Marketplace Medicine,* for an extensive discussion of the role of religious beliefs and practices in healing.

31. Ibid., 29.

32. Anthony Allen, "Healing through Medicine, Counseling, and Prayer: A Congregation-Based Ministry," monograph (n.p., n.d.), 7.

33. Cassell, *The Healer's Art.*

34. Michael Balint, *The Doctor, the Patient, and Illness* (London: International University Press, 1957).

35. Edmund Pellegrino, "Religion and Sources of Medical Morality and Healing," *New York State Journal of Medicine* (December 1981): 1863.

36. Ibid.

37. Arnold S. Relman, "Holistic Medicine," *New England Journal of Medicine* (8 February 1979): 313.

9 · The Pastor, Physician, and Nurse as Healers

1. Reginald Brightman, "Healing and the Minister," in *Religion and Medicine,* ed. Crowlesmith, 137.

2. For a further discussion see A. R. Evans, *The Healing Church*, forthcoming companion volume to *Redeeming Marketplace Medicine*, and John Crowlesmith, ed., *Religion and Medicine*, who discusses Weatherhead's writing on odic force.

3. Leslie Weatherhead, "Present-Day Non-Medical Methods of Healing," in *Religion and Medicine*, ed. Crowlesmith, 56.

4. Robert A. Lambourne, "The Healing Ministry of the Church" (lecture notes presented at University of Birmingham, Birmingham, England, n.d.), 1.

5. Melvyn Thompson, *Cancer and the God of Love* (London: SCM Press, 1976).

6. David Castle, *The Spiritual Checkup* (Newell, Iowa: Bireline, 1985).

7. Mark Siegler, "The Doctor-Patient Encounter and Its Relationship to Theories of Health and Disease," 629.

8. Dennis O'Leary, "No, but They Should Be in Charge," *Washington Post*, 5 June 1983, C8.

9. Tournier, *A Doctor's Casebook*, 216.

10. Ibid., 215.

11. Jamie Harrison and Robert Innes, *Medical Vocation and Generation X* (Cambridge: Grove Books Limited, 1997), 6.

12. Ibid., 9.

13. Pellegrino, "The Healing Relationship," 22–23.

14. Edmund Pellegrino, "Medicine of the Family and the Family of Medicine," *Urban Health* 8, no. 10 (December 1981): 235–43.

15. William F. May, *The Physician's Covenant: Images of the Healer in Medical Ethics* (Philadelphia: Westminster Press, 1983). This sounds very similar to William F. May's description of the covenant model.

16. Edmund Pellegrino, "Medical Economics and Medical Ethics: Points of Conflict and Reconciliation," *Journal of Medical Association of Georgia* 69 (March 1980): 174–83.

17. Larry Dossey, *Healing Words: The Power of Prayer and the Practice of Medicine* (San Francisco: Harper, 1993), 135–36.

18. Pellegrino, "Medicine of the Family and the Family of Medicine," 6.

19. Ibid., 5.

20. Pellegrino and Thomasma, *A Philosophical Basis of Medical Practice*, 216.

21. Richard Selzer quoted by Pellegrino in commencement address.

22. Eric Cassell, interview with the author, New York City, 21 April 1983.

23. Eric Cassell, "The Organ's Disease, the Man's Illness and the Healer's Art," *Hastings Center Report* 6 (April 1976): 29.

24. Cassell, *The Healer's Art*, 138.

25. Barth, *Church Dogmatics*, 361.

26. Tournier, *A Doctor's Casebook*, 176.

27. Eric Cassell, "Death and the Physician," *Commentary* (June 1969): 78. How prophetic are these words of three decades ago.

28. Eric Cassell, "The Physician and the Dying Patient," in *Cancer, Stress, and Death*, ed. Jean Tache, Hans Selye, and Stacey B. Day (New York: Plenum Medical Book Co., 1979), 706.

29. Ibid., 707.

30. Eric Cassell, "Learning to Die," *Bulletin of the New York Academy of Medicine* 49 (December 1973): 1116.

31. Cassell, "The Physician and the Dying Patient," 718.

32. Eric Cassell, "Telling the Truth to the Dying Patient," in *Cancer, Stress, and Death*, 122.

33. Eric Cassell, "Autonomy and Ethics in Action," *New England Journal of Medicine* 297 (11 August 1977): 333.

34. Cassell, "Learning to Die," 1117.

35. Ibid., 1118.

36. Cassell, interview with the author, 21 April 1983.

37. See W. F. May, *The Physician's Covenant*, for an excellent critique of the contract model.

38. Kass, "Regarding the End of Medicine," 24.

39. National Center for Health Statistics (www.hcfa.gov), May 1997.

40. John T. Tierney and William J. Waters, "The Evolution of Health Planning," *New England Journal of Medicine* 308, no. 2 (13 January 1983): 95–97.

41. Ruth Zerner (address at Lehman College, Department of Nursing, Bronx, New York, 25 May 1995).

42. Shirlee Passau-Buck with Edward Magruder Jones, *Male Ordered Health Care: The Inequities of Women* (Staten Island: Power Publications, 1994), 54. Only 6 percent of nurses are male; on the other hand, fewer than 25 percent of physicians are female. Ibid., 41.

43. Adeline R. Falk Rafael, "Power and Caring: A Dialectic in Nursing," *Advances in Nursing Science* (September 1996): 19(1), 3(15). The articles referred to in notes 43–61 are Web site referenced.

44. Passau-Buck, *Male Ordered Health Care*, 54.

45. Ibid., 32.

46. Jane Salvage, "What's Happening to Nursing?" *British Medical Journal* 311, no. 7000 (29 July 1995): 274.

47. Ibid., 304.

48. Colburn, "Nurses' Jobs Are Changing or Disappearing," 7–8.

49. Alison L. Kitson, "Does Nursing Have a Future?" *British Medical Journal* (21 December 1996): 313(7072), 1647(5).

50. Susan Warner Salmond, "Delivery-of-Care Systems Using Clinical Nursing Assistants: Making It Work," *Nursing Administration Quarterly* 21, no. 2 (winter 1997): 74(11); available from Health Reference Center Database, Medical Center Library, Medical Center at Princeton, New Jersey, unnumbered.

51. Linda McGillis Hall, "Staff Mix Models: Complementary or Substitution Roles for Nurses," *Nursing Administration Quarterly* 21, no. 2 (winter 1997): 31(9); available from Health Reference Center Database, Medical Center Library, Medical Center at Princeton, New Jersey, unnumbered.

52. Ibid.

53. Ibid.

54. Ibid.

55. Ibid.

56. Ibid.

57. Ibid.

58. Ibid.

59. Margretta Madden Styles, "Nursing in the Years to Come," *World Health* 47, no. 5 (September–October 1994): 26(2); available from Health Reference Center Database, Medical Center Library, Medical Center at Princeton, New Jersey, unnumbered.

60. Virginia Trotter Betts, "Nursing's Agenda for Health Care Reform: Policy, Politics, and Power through Professional Leadership," *Nursing Administration Quarterly* 20, no. 3 (spring 1996): 1(8); available from Health Reference Center Database, Medical Center Library, Medical Center at Princeton, New Jersey, unnumbered.

61. Roy L. Simpson, "The 21st Century Nurse Executive," *Nursing Administration Quarterly* 20, no. 2 (winter 1996): 85(4); available from Health Reference Center Database, Medical Center Library, Medical Center at Princeton, New Jersey, unnumbered.

62. Institute of Medicine, Committee on Improving the Patient Record, *The Computer-Based Patient Record: An Essential Technology for Health Care*, ed. Richard S. Dick and Elaine B. Steen (Washington, D.C.: National Academy Press, 1991).

63. Constance Sumner, "Recognizing and Responding to Spiritual Distress," *American Journal of Nursing* 98, no. 1 (Jan. 1998): 29.

64. Ibid.

65. Ibid., 28.

66. Annette Swackhamer, "It's Time to Broaden Our Practice," *RN* (January 1995): 58(1), 49(3).

10. THE COLLABORATION OF HEALERS

1. Frost, *Christian Healing*, 187.

2. See Emile Cailliet, *The Christian Approach to Culture* (New York: Abingdon-Cokesbury Press, 1953), especially chapter 18, for an explanation of the place of theology in modern culture and philosophy.

3. Pellegrino and Thomasma, *A Philosophical Basis of Medical Practice*, 80–81.

4. Ibid., 141.

5. Pellegrino, "Religion and Sources of Medical Morality and Healing," 1859.

6. Ibid., 1862.

7. Ibid.

8. Ibid., 1863.

9. Edmund Pellegrino, "Beyond Bioethics: The Christian Obligations of Christian Physicians" (lecture presented at Marquette University, Milwaukee, Wisconsin, March 1981), photocopy, 6.

10. Pellegrino, "Religion and Sources of Medical Morality and Healing," 1862.

11. Edmund Pellegrino, "Medicine, History, and the Idea of Man," *Annals of Political and Social Science* 346 (March 1963): 9–20.

12. Edmund Pellegrino, "The Necessity, Promise and Dangers of Human Experimentation in Experiments with Man," in *World Council Studies* 6 (New York: Friendship Press, 1969), 50.

13. Pellegrino, "Medicine, Philosophy, and Man's Infirmity," in *Conditio Humana*, ed. Walter von Beyer and Richard M. Griffith (New York: Springer Verlag, 1966), 281.

14. Ibid., 1863.

15. Edmund Pellegrino, "The Ethics of Nursing Research: Some Special Aspects," *Ethical Dimensions of Nursing Research*, Proceedings of the First Annual Scholarly Nursing Leadership Conference (University of Maryland School of Nursing, Baltimore, Maryland, 1980), 2.

16. Pellegrino and Thomasma, "Medicine as a Science of Action," 238.

17. Ibid.

18. Pellegrino, "Religion and Sources of Medical Morality and Healing."

19. Pellegrino, "Medicine, Philosophy, and Man's Infirmity," 281.

20. Pellegrino, "Beyond Bioethics," 8.

21. Ibid., 12.

22. Ibid., 17.

23. Ibid., 20.

24. Maddocks, *The Christian Healing Ministry*, 163.

25. Pattison, *Alive and Kicking*, 148.

26. Crowlesmith, *Religion and Medicine*, 174.

27. Ibid., 166–74.

28. Elisabeth McSherry, "Clergy-Physician, Co-Providers in New National Health Policy," *Lycoming Medical Society Journal* (May–June 1983): 2.

29. W. J. Kimber, *The Healing Church* (London: SPCK, 1962).

30. Niedermeyer, *Compendium of Pastoral Medicine*, 12.

Conclusion

1. Henri Nouwen, *Wounded Healer: Ministry in Contemporary Society* (Garden City, N.Y.: Doubleday, 1972).

2. In Bonhoeffer's book now titled *Cost of Discipleship*. In the new edition due in 1998–99 it will be called simply *Discipleship* since, as Bonhoeffer scholar Ruth Zerner points out, the phrase "cost of discipleship" never appears in the book as such.

3. Roland Miller, "Christ the Healer," in *Health and Healing: Ministry of the Church*, ed. Henry Lettermann (Chicago: Wheat Ridge Foundation, 1980), 35.

4. Jonathan Sacks, *Risks for Peace, Faith in the Future* (Macon, Ga.: Mercer University Press, 1997).

5. Gustavo Gutiérrez, *Theology of Liberation: History, Politics, & Salvation* (Maryknoll, N.Y.: Orbis Books, 1973).

6. Edmund Pellegrino, Proceedings of the Second International Conference organized by the Pontifical Commission for the Apostolate of Health Care Workers (10–12 November 1988), 2.

7. Quote by Gilbert Keith Chesterton, British writer (1874–1936).

Index

addiction, 24, 35, 42–43, 45, 120–21, 135, 159
Advocate Health Care, 14
AIDS, 31–32, 42, 131
allopathic medicine. *See* medical model
American Holistic Nurses Association, 151
American Medical Association, 158
Ananias and Sapphira, 83
anointing, 129–30. *See also* sacrament of healing
Aquinas, Thomas, 71, 167
Aristotle, 59, 62, 167
Asclepius, 34, 143
Augustine, 71, 111–12, 114

Balint, Michael, 129
Barth, Karl, 77, 141
Bethel Baptist Wholistic Health Center, 128
Blue Cross/Blue Shield, 11, 20
Bonhoeffer, Dietrich, 73, 166
Boorse, Christopher, 62, 76–77
British Medical Association, 158

Callahan, Daniel, 20, 33
Carlson, Rick, 48
Carter Center, 163
Cassell, Eric: views of death, 142–45; views of health, 84; views of pastor, 152–60; views of patient, 121–22, 129; views of physician, 135, 137, 140–45
Centers for Disease Control, 33, 42
chaplain, hospital, 96, 155–56
Chisholm, Brock, 33
Chow, Effie Poy Yew, 127
Christian Medical Commission (Sub Unit on Health), World Council of Christ's

healing ministry. *See* Jesus' healing ministry; Jesus' healing miracles
Christian Medical Society, 158
Christians, as healers, 165–70
churches, 63
Churches' Council for Health and Healing, 157
church fathers, 83, 94–95, 112
Clement of Alexandria, 83, 95
clinical pastoral education (CPE), 53, 163
Clinton health care reform, 7, 19
Coggan, Donald, 90
Coles, Robert, 160
Columbia Presbyterian Medical Center, 40, 52
Community of Caring, 160
courage, definition of, 69, 101, 126, 131, 167
Cousins, Norman, 123, 126
Cyprian, 83

death: causes of, 39–40, 175 n. 36; meaning in, 48, 79, 156; patient and, 26, 35, 143–45; physicians' views, 26, 35, 37, 142–45, 160; salvation and, 75, 81, 90; sin and, 80, 83
Department of Health and Social Service, 32
disease: anthropological views, 31–32; caused by, 21–22, 33; definition, 31, 60, 76–77; health reduced to absence of, 31–36, 58–59, 72–73; medical model's definition (*see* medical model); as organic, 24–25, 27; responsibility for, 23, 40, 43. *See also* illness; sickness
dualism, 35, 43, 69, 73, 133, 153, 155, 160

187